To All The Nations

To All The Nations
The Billy Graham Story

John Pollock

1817

A Ruth Graham Dienert Book

Harper & Row, Publishers, San Francisco
Cambridge, Hagerstown, New York, Philadelphia
London, Mexico City, São Paulo, Singapore, Sydney

This work incorporates material included in
BILLY GRAHAM: *Evangelist to the World* and
BILLY GRAHAM: *The Authorized Biography*, both by
John Pollock.

TO ALL THE NATIONS: *The Billy Graham Story.*
Copyright © 1985 by Worldwide Publications. All rights
reserved. Printed in the United States of America. No part of this
book may be used or reproduced in any manner whatsoever
without written permission except in the case of brief
quotations embodied in critical articles and reviews. For
information Address Harper & Row, Publishers, Inc., 10 East 53rd
Street, New York, NY 10022. Published simultaneously in Canada
by Fitzhenry & Whiteside, Limited, Toronto.

FIRST EDITION

Library of Congress Cataloging in Publication Data

Pollock, John Charles.
    To all the nations.

    Includes index.
    1. Graham, Billy, 1918–   .   2. Evangelists—
United States—Biography.   I. Title.
BV3785.G69P64   1985   269'.2'0924[B]   84-48230
ISBN 0-06-066656-0

85 86 87 88 89 10 9 8 7 6 5 4 3 2

Contents

Preface

By any reckoning, Billy Graham is one of the major religious figures of the twentieth-century.

He has addressed more than 90 million people face to face, while countless millions have seen and heard him on television and radio. Nearly two million persons have come forward as enquirers at his crusade meetings, and evidence from all over the world shows that a large number found this the beginning or deepening of their Christian life. Yet Billy Graham is far more than an evangelist and has had a profound influence on the Christianity of our time.

There is a need for an authoritative but reasonably short account, featuring the highlights of his life and work so far, especially as the authorized biography of 1966 is no longer in print. This told of his first forty-seven years. The time has not come to attempt an entirely fresh, definitive work, so I have abridged my earlier book to form Part One of the present. I have made corrections, inserted fresh evidence where necessary, and have updated the perspective: for instance I am deeply grateful to Her Majesty Queen Elizabeth the Queen Mother for graciously allowing me to quote the letter written to Billy Graham on her behalf in 1954, which in the earlier book I gave as from 'a greatly loved national figure.'

The middle years of an active contemporary are less absorbing to readers than his rise to fame or his recent work. I have dealt more briefly with the period 1960–1976, especially as this was described very fully in my second volume of authorized biography, *Billy Graham: Evangelist to the World* (1979), which is easily obtainable. I provide references to the chapters from which I have digested and updated extracts, and any reader wanting to study Graham's life, methods and ministry in greater detail should refer to that book, which I cite as *Evangelist to the World*. I am grateful to Harper and Row, publishers (New York, San Francisco, London) for their kind permission to use this material.

The years since 1977 are of greatest interest. I have picked out the highlights but have dealt at length with his controversial visit to Moscow in 1982, one of the most influential episodes of his career.

Once again, this book is based primarily on the private papers of Billy Graham and on tape-recorded evidence of a very large number of witnesses, interviewed throughout the world.

It would be impossible to thank by name all those who have helped. I am grateful to them all, but wish to thank particularly Billy Graham himself, for inviting me to study his private papers and for his encouragement throughout the work. I wish to thank the Billy Graham Evangelist Association and its President, Mr Allan C. Emery, Jr, for making possible the research and writing. All the Team and members everywhere were extremely helpful but I owe a big word of thanks to Dr Walter M. Smyth, Vice-President International Ministries; to Dr Alexander S. Haraszti, Dr Graham's Personal Representative for Eastern European Affairs, and Dr John N. Akers; and to the staff at Minneapolis, specially Mr George M. Wilson, Executive Vice-President, and Mrs Esther La Dow, his private Secretary, and her splendid team of transcribers: co-ordinated by Mrs Anna Hultquist and Mrs Sandy Malley and typed by them and other members of the secretarial staff.

Finally I would like to thank Mrs J. E. Williams for her skilled typing of the manuscript: the fourteenth book on which we have worked together. And a special word of thanks for my ever patient publisher, John Hunt, and my editor, Debbie Thorpe.

John Pollock

Part One
1918–1959

1

Sunshine in the South

William Cook Graham, a Confederate veteran with a bullet in his leg, who died in 1910 at the age of sixty, had a patriarchal beard and a large family, but nothing else Biblical about him. He drank, he swore, he neglected his farm and would not pay his debts.

He had been born at Fort Mill in York District, and after the Civil War bought the land a few miles away near Charlotte, North Carolina, which he left to two of his sons, William Franklin and Clyde. Together they built up a three-hundred-acre dairy farm of rich red soil, with woods and streams and gently rolling contours, and delivered milk in the city.

William Franklin Graham married Morrow Coffey of Steele Creek near Charlotte in 1916. Their eldest son, William Franklin Graham, Jr, Billy Frank to his family, was born in the frame farmhouse on November 7, 1918, three days before his father's thirtieth birthday and four before the Armistice.

All four of Billy Graham's grandparents were descended from the Scots-Irish pioneers who settled in the Carolinas before the Revolution. His mother's father, Ben Coffey, had fair hair and blue eyes (like his grandson) and the tall, clean-limbed, strong-jawed physique immortalized in the North Carolina monument at Gettysburg, where he fell badly wounded. A one-legged, one-eyed veteran, he was a farmer of intelligence, spirit and sterling honesty, with a tenacious memory and a love for Scripture and literature which he imparted to his daughters.

In the frame farmhouse and then in the red brick home nearby which the Grahams built when Billy was ten, with its pillared porch, paved paths, and shade of oaks and cedars, Morrow Coffey Graham kept the books, did the

11

cooking and housework and chopped the wood, with the aid of Suzie, her black maid. A blend of determination with gentleness and affection won for Morrow the complete devotion of her two sons and two daughters: Billy Frank, Catherine, Melvin, and Jean, who was fourteen years younger than Billy.

Frank Graham, was an equally strong character. Six feet two, dark haired with a fine bass voice, he was a farmer through and through. In early manhood he had experienced a religious conversion but his faith had lost urgency, though it remained the foundation of his integrity. Straight as his back in business dealings, he was adored and a little feared by the farm hands and his children. His scanty eduction was offset by shrewdness and a lively curiosity; he had a dry wit and a warm and generous nature, kept in close control because agricultural bankruptcies were frequent in the Carolinas. His one indulgence was the smoking of large cigars. He scorned relaxation and hated travel. His world was the south – placid, sunny, but smarting from the Civil War and the economic depression and poverty which it had left.

The Graham farm was comparatively prosperous. Billy Frank's hero was the foreman, Reese Brown, an army sergeant in World War I, a splendid black who could hold down a bull to be dehorned, had a wide range of skills, was tireless, efficient and trustworthy. Billy crammed down Mrs Brown's delicious buttermilk bread, the Brown children were his playmates and Reese taught him to milk and herd.

Billy was a bit too prankish to be of much use at first. High spirits and a love of adventure frequently cost him a taste of his father's belt, or his mother's long hickory switch: such discipline was normal and expected. 'Billy was rowdy, mischievous,' recalls an older cousin, 'but on the other hand, he was soft and gentle and loving and understanding. He was a very sweet, likeable person.' His parents were strict but fair, and the house was full of laughter.

Billy Graham's early education was almost as poor as Abraham Lincoln's, a primary reason being the low level of teaching; yet if the teaching had been better he would have made little use of it, for by the age of eleven he reckoned to have horse-sense enough for a future farmer, an attitude slightly abetted by his father, stoutly resisted by his mother.

His chief interest was baseball. He had been taught the game early by the McMakins, three sons of the share-cropper on his father's farm, a red-headed man of high temper but strict Christian principles, who had once been a Southern champion bicycle racer. Billy's keenness for baseball was not matched by his skill. He barely made the Sharon High School team as a first baseman, and though he dreamed of being a professional, the dream died before he left high school. Baseball influenced him most by inter-fering with his studies. The one redeeming feature of Billy's early intellectual life was an exceptional love of reading history books; by the time he was fourteen he had read about a hundred.

When Billy was small, Sunday was rather like an old Scottish Sabbath, its highlights the five-mile drive by automobile to the small Associate Reformed Presbyterian Church, which sang only metrical psalms, in Charlotte, a city then rated the most church-going in America.

He never thought of his parents as particularly religious. Then, when Billy was about fifteen, his mother joined a Bible class at the urging of her sister. Her husband remained indifferent. His energies were absorbed by the farm, especially since he had recently lost his savings in the bank failures of 1933.

Three weeks after she joined the Bible class Frank Graham's head was smashed by a flying stick of wood from the mechanical saw. The surgeons believed he would die. Mrs Graham, after calling her Christian friends to pray, went up to her bedroom 'and just laid hold of the Lord. I got up with the assurance that God heard my prayer.' Both the Grahams believed that in Frank's accident and full recovery 'the Lord really spoke to us.' They gave more time for Bible study and prayer, and she read to the children devotional books.

The adolescent Billy Frank 'thought it all hogwash.' He was in confused, mild and barely acknowledged revolt,

13

though his chief wildness was to borrow his father's car 'and drive it as fast as I could get it to go,' turning curves on two wheels, and racing other boys on the near-empty roads of North Carolina. 'Once I got the car stuck in the mud, and I had to call my father. He was more angry than I had ever seen him. He had to get mules to come and pull it out.'

Physically Billy Graham developed fast, like most Southern country boys. At high school he was much the ladies' man, with his height, wavy blond hair, blue eyes and tanned skin, his neat clothes and fancy ties. He was in and out of love, sometimes dating two girls successively the same night, but his parents expected their children 'to be clean and never doubted that we would be. They trusted us and made us want to live up to their confidence.'

Farm labour gave him the needed release of physical energy. Every day he was milking before dawn, fast and smoothly; then he helped pour the Holstein, Guernsey and Jersey milk into the big mixer before bottling. From school he hurried back to the afternoon milking. He revelled in sweat and exertion, whether cleaning out cow stalls, forking manure or pitching hay.

In May 1934 Frank Graham lent a pasture to some thirty local businessmen who wanted to devote a day of prayer for Charlotte, having planned an evangelistic campaign despite the indifference of the ministers. During that day of prayer on the Graham land their leader prayed – as Frank Graham would often recall between Billy's rise to fame in 1949 and his own death in 1962 – that 'out of Charlotte the Lord would raise up someone to preach the Gospel to the ends of the earth.'

The businessmen next erected in the city a large 'tabernacle' of raw pine on a steel frame, where for eleven weeks from September 1934 a renowned, fiery Southern evangelist named Mordecai Fowler Ham, and his song leader, Walter Ramsay, shattered the complacency of church-going Charlotte.

Ham, who was then pastor of First Baptist Church, Oklahoma, charged full-tilt at scandals and prejudices and was a mighty protagonist for Prohibition. Despite his old Southern courtesy he tended to 'skin the ministers,' as his phrase was, and cared not at all that Charlotte's most powerful clergy opposed, or that newspapers attacked him. His passionate preaching left hearers with an overwhelming realization that Christ was alive.

The Frank Grahams did not attend the Ham campaign's first week or ten days – possibly because of the tabernacle's distance and their minister's guarded neutrality toward Ham. Some neighbours then took them. After that 'we couldn't stay away.'

Billy Graham, too old to be ordered to attend, was 'definitely antagonistic,' until the Ham-Ramsey campaign exploded new controversy when Ham flung at his audience a charge of fornication among the students at the Central High School. Infuriated students marched on the tabernacle, the newspapers featured the sensation, and Billy Graham was intrigued.

Albert McMakin, the second of the sharecropper's sons, now twenty-four and newly married, had been attending the campaign regularly because a few months earlier, at one of the small preparatory meetings he had discovered that an upright life was not enough. He filled his old truck with folk from the Graham neighbourhood, both whites and blacks, and telling Billy that Ham was no 'cissy' but a fighting preacher, he invited him to drive it to the meetings.

They sat at the back of the largest crowd Billy had ever seen. Far away up the 'sawdust trail' of wood shavings sat the choir, and when vigorous, white-haired Mordecai Ham began to preach, Billy was 'spellbound,' as he wrote thirty years later. 'Each listener became deeply involved with the evangelist, who had an almost embarrassing way of describing your sins and shortcomings and of demanding, on pain of divine judgment, that you mend your ways. As I listened, I began to have thoughts I had never known before.'

That night in the room he shared with Melvin, Billy Graham gazed at the full moon and felt 'a kind of stirring in my breast that was both pleasant and scary. Next night all my father's mules and horses could not have kept me away from the meetings.'

His sixteenth birthday passed. Albert McMakin detected

15

that Billy's self-righteousness was crumbling. Ham had a habit of pointing his finger. His analysis cut so close to the bone that once Billy ducked behind the hat of the woman in front, and to escape the accusing finger applied for a place in the choir, though he could not carry a tune and his vocal efforts in the bath were a merriment to all the Grahams. He was accepted and found himself next to Grady Wilson, a casual acquaintance from another school.

The manoeuvre was futile. By now Billy had 'a tremendous conviction that I must commit myself. I'm sure,' he recalls, 'the Lord did speak to me about certain things in my life. I'm certain of that. But I cannot remember what they were. But I do remember a great sense of burden that I was a sinner before God and had a great fear of hell and judgment.'

The more he struggled to assert his own goodness the heavier grew his burden. He had no doubt now in his mind that Christ had died on the Cross to bear the sins of Billy Graham; and each night the conviction grew that Christ, whose Resurrection he had never doubted in theory, was actually alive, wanting to take away the burden, and in its place to bring Himself to be Saviour and Friend, if only Billy would commit himself unreservedly. Billy was far less conscious of Mordecai Ham than of Christ. Yet the price of Christ's friendship would be total surrender for a life-long discipleship; Billy would no longer be his own master. That price he was not yet prepared to pay. When Ham invited those who would accept Christ to move toward the pulpit in an act of witness and definition, Billy Graham stayed in his seat.

The inward struggle continued, at school desk, in the gymnasium at basketball, in the cowbarn milking. He did not tell his parents ('We suspected, and we were hoping and praying'), but talked with a first cousin, Crook Stafford, who encouraged him to go forward although Crook had not yet done so himself. Billy moved again next night and sat near the front. Ham's smile seemed consciously directed; Billy, quite wrongly, was certain Ham knew about him and quoted specially for him, 'God commendeth His love toward us in that while we were yet sinners, Christ died for us.'

16

Ham made the appeal. Billy heard the choir sing, 'Just as I am, without one plea,' verse by verse, as people gathered round the pulpit. Billy stayed in his seat, his conscience wrestling with his will. The choir began 'Almost persuaded, Christ to believe.' Billy could stand it no longer and went forward.

'It was not just the technique of walking forward in a Southern revival meeting. It was Christ. I was conscious of Him.'

A short man with dark hair and eyes approached, an English-born tailor whom Billy knew and liked, and they talked and had a prayer. Billy had a 'deep sense of peace and joy,' but around him many were in tears and he worried a bit because he felt so matter-of-fact. His father came across, threw his arms round him and thanked God for his decision.

That night Billy Graham walked upstairs past the old family clock ticking loudly the time, day and month, and undressed in the dark because Melvin was already asleep. The moon rode high again and Billy looked out across his father's land, then lay for hours unemotionally checking over in the context of his adolescent world what should be the attitudes of a fellow who belonged to Christ. He drifted into sleep content and at peace, with just a grain of doubt: 'I wonder if this will last?'

2

The Eighteenth Green

The Florida Bible Institute's elegant cream-coloured building in Spanish style at Temple Terrace, near Tampa, faced the eighteenth tee of a golf course. It had been a country club, picked up for a song at the height of the Depression by the Founder, Dr W. T. Watson. In 1937 the Institute had thirty men and forty women students. The remainder of the rooms were used as a hotel and Bible conference centre.

The Graham family drove up in a new Plymouth on a February morning in 1937 to place Billy at the school. In the two and a quarter years since the Ham mission he had grown as a Christian; he still recalls giving his first faltering testimony, in the small jail at Monroe, North Carolina, where he had gone with a young evangelist, Jimmy Johnson, who did not regard him as a candidate for fame: 'He was a typical, unpredictable, gangling tall young man,' but with great personality and very likeable. Billy had no firm ideas for a career, except that he no longer wished to be a farmer, but he wanted to continue education beyond high school.

His parents' first choice was Bob Jones College, then at Cleveland, Tennessee, because they admired several men it had produced. Following a summer in which Billy and his great friend Grady Wilson worked as Fuller Brush salesmen and Billy's sales topped the whole list, the two boys entered Bob Jones College in the fall of 1936, shortly before Billy's eighteenth birthday.

Neither the college nor the climate suited him. Billy was soon unhappy. Two bouts of flu during the Christmas vacation and the start of his respiratory troubles, increased his reluctance to return. The physician prescribed sunshine. During a family holiday with Mrs Graham's sister in

Florida they heard about the Bible Institute. Billy finished the Bob Jones semester with Dr Bob's ominous words in his ears: 'Billy, if you leave and throw your life away at a little country Bible School, the chances are you'll never be heard of. At best all you could amount to would be a poor country Baptist preacher somewhere out in the sticks.'

At Temple Terrace Billy Graham burgeoned in the freedom and family spirit, the sunshine and scenery. The school was too small for baseball, though convenient for watching (through a hole in the fence) the big league training sessions. There were tennis and volley ball and the Hillsboro River for swimming and canoeing. On the golf course Billy began to caddy, then to play. Billy worked to be like the other students though his father paid the modest fees, and as an outlet for his unceasing energy. He sought grass cutting, hedge trimming and jobs to develop his wiry strength; and dishwashing: Billy claimed to wash so fast that he could keep four girls busy.

With his natty clothes, suits regularly sent to the cleaners, bright bow ties for the evenings, Billy Graham was a favourite. A good fellow to have around: vital, generous, clean-limbed, clear-eyed. Yet he was aimless, lacking serious application to lectures or study.

At an ordinary school these virtues and defects might have left him a charming incompetent. However, the Florida Bible Institute (now Trinity College, Clearwater) put an exceptional emphasis on individual instruction; the faculty worked from the belief that the latent possibilities of each student must be fostered: that the Holy Spirit, if allowed to operate in His own time and way, could make of a man what He would. And the dean, John Minder, with his humorous eyes and endless patience, applied this principle to Graham.

Having heard Graham give his testimony outside the dog track at Sulphur Springs, Minder invited him to stay at the little conference centre he had developed on the shores of Lake Swan near Melrose in northern Florida, during the Easter vacation of 1937. On Easter Sunday evening they drove to Palatka above the broad St John's River to call on Minder's close friend Cecil Underwood, an interior

19

decorator who was a Baptist preacher. They found him setting out to supply a pulpit at the nearby country community of Bostick. In the car Underwood suggested Minder might preach. Minder replied: 'Billy's preaching tonight.'

'No, sir,' said a horrified Billy, 'I've never preached before.'

'Well, you are preaching tonight,' said Minder. 'When you run out, I'll take over.'

Billy had secretly prepared and practised four sermons on themes taken from a famous Baptist preacher, each to last forty-five minutes.

They drew up at the clapboard church, stepped through the beagles and hounds that had accompanied their masters, and joined a congregation of twenty-five or thirty cowboys and ranchers. The song leader, a man of odd jobs from junk collecting to fishing, led off in a raucous marching hymn, pausing occasionally to spit tobacco juice into the boiler. Underwood introduced Billy, whose knees knocked and palms and brow were sticky. Billy began loud and fast, and worked through all four sermons in eight minutes. But Underwood noted that 'his delivery was impressive, even that first sermon, because of his sincerity.'

Back at Temple Terrace, Minder asked Billy to preach to the young people at Tampa Gospel Tabernacle, of which Minder was pastor. That night Billy could scarcely sleep. He studied, prayed and sweated, and next morning crept out for a practice preach to the squirrels and rabbits. Sunday evening left Billy sure he would never make a preacher. His audience, however, so appreciated this dramatic, forceful youth that before the summer semester was over, Minder invited him to take charge of the young people's department.

By early 1938, when Graham had been a year at Temple Terrace and was nineteen, he was still an overgrown undisciplined boy without purpose. Three major upheavals turned him into a man of overriding purpose and intense conviction.

Two Christians whom he had admired were accused of

serious moral defections. Billy was shaken. He determined that nothing should ever be allowed in his life, known or unknown, that could harm the name of Christ. Furthermore, he realized that this could happen unless he took his vocation as a Christian seriously.

An even stronger influence began to shape him. Temple Terrace had become a vacation attraction to prominent evangelicals from North and South. Billy had the inestimable benefit of rubbing the shoulders (or at least wiping the boots) of the great. He listened attentively as they discoursed on the decline of religion in America – church budgets low, church buildings emptying, church preaching blunted and confused. These old stalwarts who had seen the fires die down had one theme: we need a prophet. We need a man to call America back to God.

A 'tremendous burden' began to weigh on Billy Graham. On walks at night across the golf course and along the open streets, laid out for housing estates never built, he faced his future. He believed he would not make a preacher: he was too poorly educated. Yet he began to sense an unmistakable call. Praying aloud as he walked the empty countryside he answered that call in Moses' words at the burning bush: 'They will not believe me, nor harken unto my voice . . . I am not eloquent.'

During these days the president's secretary, Brunette Brock, would often say, 'Billy, God has called you to preach.' In the night walks alone he tussled with excuses. His indifferent background might indeed keep him a mediocre preacher 'somewhere out in the sticks.' Yet any sacrifice appeared trivial beside Christ's sufferings or the world's needs. As for eloquence, the Lord had told Moses, 'Go, and I will be with thy mouth, and teach thee what thou shalt say.' Billy hesitated because for him the call was absolute. If he accepted, he must henceforth have no other ambition, no other occupation but the proclaiming of God's message, everywhere, to everybody, always.

One night in March 1938 Billy Graham returned from his walk and reached the eighteenth green immediately before the school's front door. 'The trees were loaded with Spanish moss, and in the moonlight it was like a fairyland.'

He sat down on the edge of the green, looking up at the moon and stars, aware of a warm breeze from the south. The tension snapped. 'I remember getting on my knees and saying "O God, if you want me to preach, I will do it."'

In the days following, 'I used to walk those empty streets in Temple Terrace praying. I would pray sometimes three or four hours at a stretch. And then,' he recalled a quarter of a century after, 'in the most unusual way I used to have the strangest glimpses of these great crowds that I now preach to.' He certainly did not see himself as the preacher, and scarcely believed great crowds would ever come together again to hear the Gospel, but the daydreams or visions flashed across his consciousness. 'I think I saw myself as participating in some way in what Billy Sunday and D. L. Moody had witnessed – big stadiums, big meetings.'

Some weeks later he faced a third upheaval: the girl whom he hoped to marry was no longer sure.

Emily Regina Cavanaugh, one class senior to Billy, was a sparkling personality, intelligent, musical, vivacious, dedicated. Billy had 'loved her from the moment I saw her.' During the summer vacation of 1937 he had proposed, by letter. In February 1938 she had accepted him. They did not expect to marry for three or four years but their friends and families rejoiced. Early in May Emily told Billy that she was again uncertain, and asked him to pray.

In a basement room, every day for a quarter of an hour, Billy would pray that they should marry – if, and only if, it were God's will. Emotional suspense bred spiritual development, for hitherto he had seldom related prayer to specific matters, as distinct from the wide sweeping vistas of the world's need; never before had he seen such answers.

Emily found herself deeper in love with Charles Massey, a senior classman whom Billy admired. Before Class Night in May 1938 each of the boys ordered from Larson the florist a twenty-five-cent corsage for his girl. Billy exclaimed: 'I'll buy a fifty-cent one. Emily must have the best.'

Emily did not wear it.

During the party she asked Billy outside. They sat on one of the swings on the riverside, and she told him gently that she was going to marry Charles.

They parted friends. Billy sought John Minder, who consoled him by the Scripture verse, 'The God of all comfort comforteth us in all our tribulation, that we may be able to comfort them which are in any trouble.' Billy bravely rejoined the social evening.

'One of two things can happen in a time like that,' comments Billy. 'You can resist and become bitter, or you can let God break you. And I determined to let God have his way.' 'Every letter he wrote home,' recalled his mother years later, 'he was heart broken; you could read that between the lines. But instead of it depressing him he turned to the Lord and the Lord sustained him. Every letter was full of that.'

Billy threw himself into his newly accepted commission to preach. 'I now had a purpose, an objective, a call. That was when the growing up began, and the discipline to study.'

At first he was forced to create most of his opportunities. 'I would take two or three students with me, or somebody that would sing, and go down on a street corner.' On Sundays he would hold seven or eight street-corner services. Once he began preaching in front of a saloon, full of alcoholics and prostitutes, on Franklin Street, in those days Tampa's worst. 'I stood right in the door, preaching to the people sitting at the bar. The bar-keeper came out and ordered me away, and I wouldn't go. He just shoved me down, and I half fell and half tripped into the wet street. I got my clothes messed up. I remembered the words of Jesus, and felt that I was suffering for Christ's sake. It was quite tactless the way I went about it, zeal with no knowledge; but those were experiences that helped develop me.'

The first time he gave the 'invitation' or altar call was at Venice on the Gulf shore, in the only church, a converted meat market. The parents of a Bible Institute girl had telephoned for a supply preacher. The morning service seemed sluggish, so Graham and his soloist spent the afternoon praying on the dirt floor of the garage at their hosts', who were out encouraging the local youths to attend. The church that evening was crowded.

Billy thought his sermon indifferent, but when he gave

the invitation, thirty-two young men and women came forward. The superintendent of the Sunday school remarked afterward, 'There's a young man who is going to be known around the world!'

Billy secured a regular invitation to the Tampa City Mission. He was made a chaplain to the trailer parks. He visited the prisoners at the Stockade. 'That's where I started my discussion groups. I had them ask me questions. A lot of them I couldn't answer, but I did it deliberately not only to help them, but to try to sharpen my mind.'

He was always seeking to educate himself. Most ministers acquire learning and then, from the superiority of pastorate or priesthood, begin to impart. Graham learned to preach while his fund of knowledge was limited. 'I had one passion, and that was to win souls. I didn't have a passion to be a great preacher; I had a passion to win souls. I'd never been trained as a public speaker. I had to learn in the best way I knew.' His stock of sermons was small, but he knew exactly what he would say. He did not write them out except in skeleton, but he practised them, even to cypress swamps and alligators. He was not perfecting a technique. 'It was all unconscious. I wasn't practising gestures; I was practising my material, learning my material. I felt I was not prepared to preach a sermon until I had practised it many, many times.'

He preached too loud. He preached too fast. He dramatized and was dubbed 'the preaching windmill', but the tramps, alcoholics, prisoners, and the northern winter visitors in the trailer parks knew what Billy meant. His aim, whether preaching or speaking with individuals, was not to promote an idea but to bring them to know the living Christ. Dedication to a cause or an idea might have hardened or narrowed Billy Graham; dedication to a Person sweetened him. The chief fault was lack of balance. He practised and prayed so hard by day that he mounted an evening pulpit worn out. His mind refused to relax at night. Light sleeping became the insomnia which has troubled him ever since.

In the summer of 1939 John Minder departed for six weeks in California, leaving Billy in charge of the Tampa

Gospel Tabernacle, where he learned the hard labour of ministry to the poor. During his last year at the Institute, while war came to Europe far away, he was in growing demand at obscure churches and chapels in different parts of Florida. With his parents' approval, he became a Southern Baptist. He was ordained in 1939 by the St John's Association at Peniel, Cecil Underwood's white-painted clapboard church under the cedar trees between Silver Lake and Lake Rosie.

In May 1940, at graduation, the class valedictorian, Vera Resue, her mind on the war and the spiritual darkness engulfing the world, and without thought of an individual, uttered words which years afterward were seen to be prophetic. At each critical epoch of the church, she said, God has 'a chosen human instrument to shine forth His light in the darkness. Men like Luther, John and Charles Wesley, Moody and others who were ordinary men, but men who heard the voice of God . . . It has been said that Luther revolutionized the world. It was not he but Christ working through him. The time is ripe for another Luther, Wesley, Moody. There is room for another name in this list.'

3

The Girl from China

A brown-haired, hazel-eyed girl of twenty, a second-year student at Wheaton College near Chicago, was in the entrance to East Blanchard Hall in the fall of 1940 when she noticed a blond fellow whom she did not know running down the steps. 'He was tall and lanky and just dashed past,' and she thought, 'There's a young man who knows where he's going!'

The father of one of her friends had told Ruth Bell to keep an eye out for a young minister and remarkable preacher called Billy Graham coming to campus, but she had not met him. Some days later she was one of a group of students meeting for prayer before going out to teach Sunday School, or for similar work. They divided into small parties in the lobby of Williston Hall and went into different rooms. 'We would take turns praying, and all of a sudden I heard a voice from the next room. I had never heard anyone pray like it before. I knew that someone was talking to God. I sensed that here was a man that knew God in a very unusual way.'

Billy Graham had entered Wheaton as a freshman. Keen for a university education he had seized an opening offered in Florida by relatives of the new president of Wheaton, V. Raymond Edman, though it would mean living in the unfamiliar world of the northern states. To work his way at college Billy had joined a senior, Johnny Streater, in running a truck, and it was Streater who effected the introduction between Billy and Ruth, in the lobby of Williston Hall outside the college cafeteria. Billy fell in love at first sight.

Ruth and Billy went together to the glee club's *Messiah* on a snowy Sunday afternoon and afterward to supper at Professor Lane's. Billy 'just could not believe anyone could be so beautiful and so sweet.' They stood a long time talking beside a tree near the college entrance. Billy wrote to his mother that this was the girl he would marry. Ruth had not fallen in love with Bill, as she always calls him; yet that very first Sunday night she knelt at her bedside in wordless prayer and 'told the Lord that if I could spend the rest of my life serving Him with Bill, I would consider it the greatest privilege imaginable.'

Ruth McCue Bell was born of Virginia parents in North China where her father, a Presbyterian surgeon, had helped develop a substantial missionary hospital despite civil wars and Japanese occupation.[1] Dr Bell described his daughter in childhood as 'an interesting mixture of deep spirituality and mischievous fun.' The second of three sisters, with a younger brother, she had spent most of her life in the Orient. At Wheaton her housemother wrote of her in 1943: 'Very attractive, beautiful to look at and excellent taste in dress. The most beautiful Christian character of any young person I have ever known. And she has the intellectual qualities to make a success in any work she would choose to undertake. She ranks very high in the qualities of poise, forcefulness, and courtesy.'

Ruth had many admirers. That first Sunday night, back at Professor Gerstung's home where he roomed, Billy Graham slumped in a chair and 'bemoaned the fact (Gerstung recalls) that he had no chance with Ruth because he had so little to commend him.'

Ruth soon thought otherwise. 'There was a seriousness about him; a depth. He was much older in every way than the other students on the campus, not just in age. He was a mature man; he was a man who knew God; he was a man who had a purpose, a dedication in life; he knew where he was going. He wanted to please God more than any man I'd ever met.' She recognized that he was a very intelligent man, though in no sense an 'egghead'. Her one reservation was that, though there was plenty of fun in his personality,

1. See: *A Foreign Devil in China*: the story of L. Nelson Bell, by John Pollock. Zondervan, Grand Rapids, 1971; Hodder and Stoughton, London, 1972.

'he was so very serious about life in general. He didn't have enough time to go to ball games. Every date we had was to a preaching service of some kind. Yet for all his terrific dedication and drive there was a winsomeness about him, and a consideration for other people, which I found very endearing.'

Love grew, but Ruth's ambition was to be a pioneer missionary in Tibet, and for this she was prepared to renounce romance. Billy, though closely interested in foreign missions, had no indication that God called him to be a missionary. He believed that Ruth was essentially a homemaker, not a pioneer, and that when she married, it would be to him. He bided his time. The Bells returned on furlough in the spring of 1941. In the summer Ruth and Billy became engaged.

Back at Wheaton Ruth again feared that to marry him would deny a clear missionary call, unless he too were bound for Tibet. He prayed, and had no leading there. Finally Billy asked her, 'Do you believe that God brought us together?' Ruth did, unquestionably. Billy pointed out that the Bible teaches that the husband is head of the wife: 'God will lead me and you will do the following.' Ruth agreed, in faith.

More than anyone Ruth broadened Graham's mind. She had no need to polish his manners or graces, as D. L. Moody's were polished by his wife, but she was cultured, travelled, with a love of art and literature. She saved his seriousness from degenerating into stuffy solemnity, and preserved from extinction the light touch, the slice of small boy. Moreover Ruth and her family, loyal Presbyterians, eased Billy Graham from his unspoken conviction that a vigorous Scriptural faith could not dwell within the great denominations; and underlined Wheaton's lesson that a strong evangelical should focus his vision on the entire horizon of Christianity.

Billy, who expected to go on to theological seminary, chose a non-theological subject as his major at Wheaton: anthropology, a new, exciting course under an able professor, Alexander Grigolia. Billy made good grades and might have made the honour roll had not his life again taken an unusual turn in the fall of 1941.

Dr Edman wished to be relieved of his part-time pastorate of the United Gospel Tabernacle of Wheaton and Glen Ellyn, a small independent church served previously by student pastors. On his recommendation the deacons offered it to Billy Graham, who was spending his vacation preaching in youth crusades in Florida.

The Tabernacle hired a small hall. Virtually no more than a preaching centre, it was the church of many students and faculty. In the words of an associate professor Graham's delivery was 'rapid, earnest, forceful, simple, a very direct approach. He had a message he wanted to get across, and it came right through without hesitation and stumbling.' There might be extravagances, mispronunciations, a touch of Mordecai Ham and the sawdust trail, but the hall was always packed. Ruth's memory, endorsed by that of Wheaton contemporaries, is that 'you weren't impressed with his earnestness, you weren't impressed by his gestures. You were impressed that there was Someone speaking to you beside Bill. There was another voice than his.'

The Tabernacle, and later his presidency of the Christian Student Council, interfered with studies, but Graham thirsted for learning. He became one of the circle of the hospitable, wealthy Professor Mortimer Lane, a much-travelled former public servant, who combined knowledge of the Bible with a gift for imparting an understanding of politics and economics. Billy became fascinated by the American political and economic scene.

After Pearl Harbor he offered himself as an Army chaplain. He was told to finish college, and his professors persuaded him not to volunteer for combat duty. As the Army required him, after graduation, to do a year at seminary or in a pastorate, he accepted one without consulting Ruth, to her considerable indignation. Western Springs was a typical semi-rural, high middle-class suburb of Chicago: straight streets, houses with unfenced lawns, and ten or more places of worship including a well-supported Methodist centre – and one mortgage-ridden Baptist church in a basement, which appointed him to be pastor immediately on graduation.

Billy and Ruth were married on Friday, August 13, 1943,

at Montreat, the Presbyterian conference centre in the mountains of North Carolina where the Bells had settled when the war prevented return to China. After a week's honeymoon in a room in a cottage at Blowing Rock, high in the Blue Ridge Mountains, the Grahams returned to Illinois and made their home in a four-room apartment in Hinsdale, a neighbouring community, since they could find no place in Western Springs. They were one block from the main line of the Burlington Railroad, and for the first week every train sounded as if it were going straight through the living room.

Billy uncomplainingly endured Ruth's early adventures in cookery, and Ruth the muddle on Billy's desk and his habit of treating the top of the bathroom door as a towel rack. They differed in temperament and in many ideas. 'If you agree on everything, there's not going to be much growth for either one,' Ruth commented long after. 'I don't think happy marriages are ever accidental. They are the result of good, hard work.' The Graham's love for one another fast grew deep and abiding.

The church people enjoyed his sermons, were amused by the loud socks and ties, gratified by Ruth's poise and smartness despite a restricted wardrobe. Billy organized house-to-house calls, sought out storekeepers, especially those that other ministers preferred not to know, and with Bob Van Kampen launched the Western Suburban Professional Men's Club, meeting over dinner seven times a winter, to which Graham personally persuaded business executives of highest rank and tightest schedules. Soon he had more than three hundred men dining to listen to an evangelistic speaker.

Billy was deepening his understanding of the importance of a pastor in the work of evangelism, but a little church in a suburb seemed trivial in the midst of a world war. He waited impatiently for his chaplaincy commission.

Then, early in October 1943, came a telephone call from Torrey Johnson, pastor of a flourishing church, professor of New Testament Greek, but best known around Chicago for his broadcasts. Billy, almost not believing his ears, heard the suggestion that his 'Village Church' take over Johnson's

Songs in the Night – forty-five minutes of preaching and singing carried live by one of Chicago's most powerful commercial stations from 10.15 pm each Sunday.

The cost would be over $100 weekly, and the station required an initial contract for thirteen weeks. The pledged income of The Village Church was $86.50 a week; yet the people raised among themselves in advance enough for five broadcasts.

Billy now flew high. In Chicago lived a Canadian-born bass baritone of thirty-seven named George Beverly Shea, famous as Christian soloist and broadcaster, especially on the American Broadcasting Company's *Club Time*, a programme of hymns. One of his own compositions, 'I'd Rather Have Jesus', was already popular. Billy went to the radio station where Shea was programme manager and announcer and received a polite brush-off from the receptionist. After turning to go out Billy thought, 'No, I've come to see him. I'm going to see him.' And he walked straight in.

Beverly Shea was gracious and guarded, Billy persistent. *Songs in the Night*, with Beverly Shea, came on the air from Western Springs in January 1944.

Young people from all over the Chicago area would hurry out after their own evening church services to see and hear Beverly Shea in person. Letters came, money came, covering not only the broacast but enabling Billy solemnly to burn the mortgage of the church in a pie plate. Billy's Southern accent, now deliberately tamed, was an immediate hit with the Yankees. And he preached in the way that was to become specially his: against a backdrop of the latest news and world events he would proclaim the urgent relevance of Christ in such manner that the listener longed to know Him. Billy urged immediate decision.

In the spring of 1944, Torrey Johnson offered an even greater opportunity.

Johnson was concerned about the hundreds of servicemen who swept into Chicago every weekend, tough, cynical, sex-starved, indifferent to God and man. On the last Saturday night of April 1944 he found an answer. He was present in First Baptist Church at Minneapolis, where a thirty-year-old businessman named George M. Wilson had organized a 'Youth for Christ Rally', in the belief that the Gospel could reach servicemen, and unchurched civilians too, if clean excitement was linked with an uncompromising Christian message. Johnson immediately formed 'Chicagoland's Youth for Christ' and booked the Orchestra Hall, with three thousand seats, next door to the USO Center, for twenty-one Saturday nights. Most of Chicago rated him foolish.

For preacher at his opening rally he chose Billy Graham. Johnson could have had any famous preacher but wished to work with the young ministers who shared his vision and had instinctive understanding of their generation. Johnson had not the slightest doubt that for an evangelistic sermon to youth, Billy Graham had no equal.

Johnson saw him 'thrilled at the prospect but dreadfully afraid he might fail.' On Saturday evening, May 20, 1944, they gathered in the stage room of Orchestra Hall. Billy paced up and down, biting his nails, palms sticky, throat dry, 'the worst fit of stage fright of my life.' They prayed together and walked onto the stage. With one consent they kept their eyes to the stalls, daring to hope that these at least would be full. They glanced higher and saw the lower balcony full too; and, to their wonder, the upper. Only the high 'peanut gallery' was thin. Someone reckoned a total of 2,800, mostly service personnel, were present.

After a swift programme of songs and instrumental music, community singing, Bible reading and prayer, Billy began to preach. Words came tumbling. 'As my nerves relaxed, I felt I was merely a mouthpiece and soon became unaware of the audience.' At the invitation to commit their lives, Billy marvelled to see forty-two people come forward, a high number for the times.

In October Graham was commissioned a second lieutenant in the United States Army, with orders to await entry to a chaplains' training course at Harvard Divinity School. Then he got mumps.

The mumps took the most virulent and painful form, his temperature raged and one night Ruth thought him dying. He was in bed six weeks, emerging thin as a lath, and thankful to go to Florida, helped by a listener's gift.

Torrey Johnson was in Florida too. At Miami, out in a fishing boat under the Florida sun which Billy so loved, Torrey outlined a plan to co-ordinate Saturday night rallies across the country, to capture and inspire American youth. Since the Army would relegate a convalescent to a desk, Billy should now resign his commission and his church, and with such funds as Johnson could raise, become the first full-time organizer and evangelist of Youth for Christ.

Billy, like Johnson, saw it as a spearhead of return to a forthright Christianity – in America, Canada, the world.

4

Geared to the Times

During 1945 Graham travelled throughout the United States and Canada, hurrying back whenever he could to Montreat, where the Grahams lived with the Bells and later in their own home next door. Their first child, Virginia (known as Gigi, Chinese for 'sister') was born in September. Billy and Ruth missed each other terribly. It was harder on the wife left behind, but a missionary childhood had prepared her for frequent goodbyes.

Graham and the Youth for Christ pioneers believed in a combination of efficient organization and daring faith. Their Saturday night rallies went in for bright solos, choirs and bands. They wore loud handpainted ties and bright suits, that all the world might know Christianity to be no dreary faith. Clothes and excitements were essentially contemporary American, but rally organizers learned to cut back on the noise and the glamour and the lights if Billy Graham were the preacher: a long musical programme meant a short sermon, 'and if I preach short we're not going to do the job of winning souls.'

The motto was 'Geared to the Times, Anchored to the Rock.' At a time when denominational leaders were convinced that the great Christian doctrines no longer might be preached with emphasis, Youth for Christ demonstrated that young men and women would respond to the unashamed proclamation of a Christ who worked miracles, shed His blood on the Cross, rose bodily from the dead, and could transform the lives of any who accepted Him. The Bible became again, not a document to be mutilated or a set of propositions to be defended, but a living Word.

Once the War ended, Torrey Johnson wished to introduce Youth for Christ to Britain and Europe. He selected Billy for his four-man team, but since they daringly decided to cross the Atlantic by air they could not obtain passages until March 1946.

They rushed through England, Scotland and Ireland in three weeks. The American's blend of seriousness and boyishness left hosts rather at a loss. They were astonished, for instance, when at the Manchester rally Billy and the soloist went to the telephone box in the interval, and preached and sung to a rally at Birkenhead over a previously booked landline.

Billy was not generally regarded as showing the greatest potential in the team. He endeared himself as 'a man of much courtesy and Christian gentlemanliness'; and whereas the others were considered a trifle blasé and know-all Americans, Billy was soaking up the British scene. 'Learning was an insatiable desire with me. I burned to learn, and I felt my limitations of schooling and background so terribly that I determined to try to do all I could through conversations, picking everything I could from everybody.'

Billy Graham fell in love with Britain. He had begun with a tendency to dismiss the clergy as neither geared to the times nor anchored to the Rock, but knew now that a genuine revival must come through the mainstream denominations. The Southerner who had scarcely met an Episcopalian began even to grasp the peculiar significance of the Church of England.

During the summer of 1946 he raised money in America and in October he was back in Britain with his own team – Cliff and Billie Barrows.

One year previously Graham had gone to Ben Lippen Bible Conference in the North Carolina mountains to address a youth night. The conference song leader had left. Graham was offered an athletic Californian, twenty-two years old and on his honeymoon. He accepted Cliff Barrows dubiously under the impression that this was a newly graduated college kid. Doubts were instantly dispersed when Cliff's skill and sunny disposition, aided by a fine voice, a trombone, and the piano playing of his wife Billie, extracted every ounce of song from a delighted audience.

Barrows, son of a farmer in the San Joaquin Valley, had

studied sacred music at college. Ordained a Baptist minister in California, Barrows spent nearly a year as an assistant pastor in Minnesota, with special responsibility for song leading and youth.

Graham had money enough for six months in Britain, provided they were frugal. Their target was not correspondingly modest: 'We are asking God for a thousand souls a month, and a thousand young people to respond to the challenge of the mission field.' The meetings began in an obscure small Welsh town called Gorseinon, where Billy and George Wilson of Minneapolis, who had come over to help set up the tour, were guests of a mining family, the two in one bed and so cold because of the national fuel rationing that they would go to bed right after the meeting with clothes on. Breakfast every morning was a tomato stuffed with bread. For a whole week they never saw meat.

Graham and the Barrows spoke in twenty-seven cities and towns of the British Isles, at 360 meetings, between October 1946 and March 1947. A David and Jonathan bond was forged. They were alike in dedication, in ability to work without stint, but Barrows was not highly strung, and no one ever saw him bite his nails. Young Cliff nursed a secret hope that he too would become an evangelist in his own right, yet he consistently pushed Graham forward. The two steadily evolved methods slightly less brash and noisy, although to the British and Irish the very idea of a song leader with a trombone was sensational. And Billy went on learning, spiritually and intellectually, from whoever he could.

At Birmingham, where in 1946 over 90 per cent of the 1,000,000 citizens were said never to attend a church regularly, adverse reports of Youth for Christ's 'showmanship' in America caused cancellation of the city hall. Ministers snubbed the organizers, and the first night of a ten-day campaign drew a paltry two or three hundred persons.

Stanley Baker, one of the ministers who had refused to help, a middle-aged Baptist, heard the telephone ring and found himself, as he wrote a week or two later, 'linked with a wounded spirit and a painted heart. He wasn't bitter, he didn't chide me; he hadn't one word of a lecture; he merely wondered . . . Within an hour I sat in Billy's hotel room . . . His was the nearest spirit to my Lord's I have ever met.' Baker at once began telephoning ministers, and Billy paid calls on some twenty. One by one they began to help. Billy moved into the Grand Hotel instead of staying on at a home in the suburbs, and several nights two or three ministers remained into the small hours praying with him for blessing on Birmingham.

Numbers rose nightly. They secured the city hall after all for a packed Saturday and Sunday, when scores came forward, young and old. The Lord Mayor hastily reissued a cancelled invitation for tea. The Bishop of Birmingham, the extreme liberal, Ernest Barnes, asked the twenty-eight-year-old Graham to address a diocesan gathering on 'Evangelism in the Twentieth Century'.

The British nation as a whole remained unaware of Graham's existence. The national press ignored him. Many evangelicals remained cautious, but an Anglican clergyman, Tom Livermore, arranged a Graham–Barrows youth campaign centred on his southeast London parish in February 1947. The worst winter for a hundred years combined with the national fuel crisis to produce an icy fog-bound church and darkened streets along which young and old stumbled through the snow. Billy, bounding up the pulpit looking to Londoners like a film star, says Livermore, 'had a tremendous appeal to the ignorant and unlettered and the rougher element of the boys and girls.' The same was true in the fog-enclosed, bomb-shattered port of Southampton, where Joe Blinco, a Methodist pastor and evangelist, felt this man 'was fresh from God; his message had a freshness about it – cleanness in the sense that a mountain might be cleaned out by the wind and the rain.'

Blinco, by origin and ministry a man of the people, also recognised Graham's social concern. It might be still naive or dogmatic, but 'Billy, from the very first time I remember him, spoke always against the background of the tragic situation in society.' And he had so strong a world vision that Blinco discounted it as American big talk, until he came to know Graham better.

37

When the tour ended with a conference of two hundred and fifty leaders in youth work, summoned by Graham to Birmingham in March, several Britons had begun to believe that Billy Graham should return for a campaign not limited to youth. They had caught a gleam which could pierce war weariness, and the defeatism, the little-mindedness which had settled on much of British religion.[1]

1. Historically it is a nice touch that the first conference organized by Graham in Britain, of 250 persons, should have been held in the city where 37 years later 11,800 clergy and lay leaders converged from all over England to hear him, on 26 January 1984.

5

Los Angeles 1949

By the summer of 1949 the thirty-year-old Graham had become much more than an evangelist to youth. Though not yet known nationally, he had a growing reputation in North America as an evangelist for 'city wide campaigns', as they were called, the phrase carrying more potential than accuracy.

He was in demand at Bible conferences. After one conference a fellow-speaker wrote to Billy: 'I do thank God for the transparency of your life and the sweetness of your spirit. No wonder he uses you so mightily, and I pray that you may ever be kept so humble and so sweet in the will of the Lord.' Billy's personal character undergirded his message; and he was already much concerned to remove the tarnish which had settled on American mass-evangelism since the great days of D. L. Moody.

Billy was also now the reluctant, if energetic, president of North Western schools, a large interdenominational Bible school, seminary and liberal arts college at Minneapolis, the pleasant city of lakes and woods and nearly half a million inhabitants in the heart of the Scandinavian region of America. Against his better judgement he had accepted the death-bed pleas of its founder, the veteran evangelical, W. B. Riley. The presidency of North Western was a diversion from evangelism. But it stretched the mind, gave Billy Graham invaluable training in finance, promotion and administration, helped teach him delegation and the moulding of a team, and how to tap the right sources of advice. It brought several colleagues who would work with him on a wider field, while Minneapolis became the natural centre for the administration of his expanding ministry. And North Western's tensions and difficulties put into his spirit the steel without which no man comes to greatness.

39

Graham now faced a date with destiny: a three week campaign in his first major city, Los Angeles, with Cliff Barrows, Bev Shea and Grady Wilson as his team, in late September 1949. 'I want to see God sweep in,' he told a somewhat hesitant committee, 'because if Los Angeles could have a great revival, the ramifications and repercussions would sweep across the entire world.' Yet when the committee accepted his conditions he was almost sorry. Billy Graham was in the thick of a spiritual battle within his own soul.

His close friend and former colleague in Youth for Christ, Charles Templeton, had become unsure of the integrity of Scripture. 'Billy, your faith is too simple,' he insisted. Billy took Templeton seriously, but the more Billy debated and read, the more confused he grew.

Could he, in the middle of the twentieth century, continue to accept the authority of the Bible? Could he, with the Apostle Paul, 'declare unto you the gospel . . . how that Christ died for our sins according to the scriptures; and that He was buried, and that He rose again according to the scriptures?' This was not loss of faith but loss of balance, yet the 'terrific pain at the base of my skull', which plagued him in the spring of 1949 and puzzled the doctors, was probably induced, as Graham suggested, by nervous tension and exhaustion.

In June the team held a ten-day campaign at the railroad city of Altoona, Pennsylvania. Local preparation had been scanty and the ministers were at each other's throats, but Billy believed the cause of failure lay in himself, his nagging uncertainties.

After Altoona Billy felt that he must decide once and for all, either to spend his life studying whether or not God had spoken, or to spend it as God's ambassador, bringing a message which he might not fully comprehend in all details until after death. Must an intellectually honest man know everything about the Bible's origins before he could use it?

Graham believed that his special gift lay in 'the invitation' to receive Christ: he was primarily a 'doorkeeper in the house of my God', helping people to enter; once entered they would be aided by others to appreciate the treasures of the house and learn more fully to serve. At a Bible conference in Michigan in July 1949 he was talking with his old Florida friend, Roy Gustafson, and became 'very, very serious. He looked at me with those piercing eyes and he said, "Roy, when I come to my invitation I sense God come on me, and I feel a power at that invitation that's peculiar."' And now might he be preaching a doubtful Gospel derived from a not wholly trustworthy Bible?

At the same conference Gustafson and another friend were with Billy when the aurora borealis lit up the sky. They began talking of the Second Advent. Suddenly Billy said, 'Oh, if somehow the Lord could use me a little bit.' They decided to have their prayer time under the stars and northern lights. In a few moments they heard a strange, muffled voice. Billy lay full-length in the wet grass with his face into the ground, praying: 'Lord, trust me to do something for You before You come!'

In the last days of August Billy and Templeton went to California as faculty members of a student conference at Forest Home, five thousand feet high in the pine-laden air of the San Bernardino Mountains behind Los Angeles. One evening, in serious discussion, a mutual friend reported a remark by Templeton: 'Poor Billy. If he goes on the way he's going he'll never do anything for God. He'll be circumscribed to a small little narrow interpretation of the Bible, and his ministry will be curtailed. As for me, I'm taking a different road.'

Templeton is sure that he never made such a remark; but whatever his actual words, these were the ones to reach Billy.

Billy was deeply disturbed and hurt. After supper, instead of attending evening service, he retired to his log cabin and read again the Bible passages concerning its authority. He recalled someone saying that the prophets used such phrases as 'the Word of the Lord came' or 'thus saith the Lord' more than two thousand times. He meditated on the attitude of Christ: 'He loved the Scriptures, quoted from them constantly, and never once intimated that they might be wrong.'

41

Billy went out in the forest and wandered up the mountain, praying as he walked, 'Lord, what shall I do? What shall be the direction of my life?' He knew he had reached a crisis. He saw that intellect alone could not resolve the question of authority. He must go beyond intellect. He thought of the faith used constantly in daily life: was it only in things of the Spirit that faith was wrong?

'So I went back and I got my Bible, and I went out in the moonlight. And I got to a stump and put the Bible on the stump, and I knelt down, and I said, "Oh, God; I cannot prove certain things, I cannot answer some of the questions Chuck is raising and some of the other people are raising, but I accept this Book by faith as the Word of God."'

Six weeks later Billy wrote from Los Angeles to his college staff at Minneapolis: 'You would have thrilled if you could have seen the great tent packed yesterday afternoon with 6,100 people and several hundred turned away, and seen the scores of people walking down the aisles from every direction accepting Christ as personal Saviour when the invitation was given.'

The committee had worked hard, all was soaked in prayer, and Billy had never seen such numbers in a city-wide campaign. In the third week, as the scheduled closing date drew near several committee men were ready to stop, well satisfied even if most of the millions who lived in the fast-moving, thrusting city and county of Los Angeles, from Hollywood to Chinatown, had not been aware of the 'canvas cathedral' or Billy Graham: others urged continuance, citing the rising interest and attendance. Right up to the Sunday afternoon Billy hesitated, for he had never previously extended a campaign. As he and Cliff prayed they decided to announce a short extension and meanwhile, like Gideon in the Book of Judges, to 'put out a fleece' – watch for a sign.

The sign came by way of a telephone call in the small hours, from Stuart Hamblen, a massive Texas cowboy, broadcaster and songwriter, in his late thirties, who was already a legend on the West Coast.

42

Stuart Hamblen was a dance band leader, a great hunter, race horse owner and gambler, and a heavy drinker. And, as he later said, 'a hypocrite': son of a Methodist preacher in Texas, he had 'left it all behind', yet he ran a children's 'Cowboy Church of the Air'.

His tiny wife, Suzy, had prayed for him for sixteen years. She had seized an opportunity to introduce him to Billy Graham shortly before the campaign began, and Stuart had taken to a fellow southerner and interviewed him on his radio chat show. He even attended with Suzy the first week, sitting in the front row feeling patronizing, and then entertained the Grahams to supper.

In the second week Billy's long finger seemed pointed right at him: 'There is somebody in this tent who is leading a double life.' Hamblen genuinely believed such remarks were deliberately aimed. After one more night he fled to the Sierras on a hunting trip, not returning until midnight on the supposed final Sunday, October 16.

With ill grace Hamblen was beside Suzy in the front row on Monday night. 'When Billy Graham got up and preached a terrific sermon, I said, Oh, that is a lot of malarky, he is lying. When they took up the collection, I said, That is a racket! When they sang some wonderful hymns, I said, That singing is lousy.' The long finger pointed again. 'There is a person here tonight who is a phoney.' Stuart Hamblen rose from the seat in a fury, shook his fist at Billy and stormed out in the middle of the sermon.

He went from bar to bar but the drinks turned sour on him. 'At last I gave up and started home, and on the way Christ spoke to me.' Hamblen fought back. He was still fighting when he stormed into the bedroom where Suzy was asleep, got her out of that bed and yelled, 'Let's pray.' They prayed; 'but I still couldn't make connections.'

About 2 am Stuart said that since Billy was the man who had upset him they would wake him. Billy answered the telephone, could hear that Stuart had been both drinking and crying, and told him to 'come right on down' to the apartment hotel where the Grahams and the Grady Wilsons shared an efficiency suite.

Stuart, with Suzy trailing behind, banged on the apartment door. It was opened by Billy in slacks and sweater. Stuart roared, 'I want you to pray for me.'

Billy replied, 'No, I'm not going to do it.' Stuart nearly knocked him down.

'Come in, Stuart,' Billy said, 'and I'll tell you why.'

Billy knew that Stuart Hamblen was like the Rich Young Ruler and refused to help him to a selfish, easy faith. At one point in their talk Billy even said, 'Go on back home. If you're not going to go all the way and let Jesus Christ be the actual Lord of every area of your life, don't ask me to pray with you, and don't waste anybody else's time.'

At last, about 5 am Stuart 'promised I would give up all that was mean and wicked in my heart.' They prayed together, 'and as I knelt by that chair I felt I was kneeling at the feet of my Jesus. "Lord," I prayed, "you're hearing a new voice this morning."'

That very day Stuart Hamblen told his radio audience that he had given his life to Christ. 'I've quit smoking and I've quit drinking. Tonight at the end of Billy's invitation, I'm going to hit the sawdust trail.' The sensation was enormous. Hundreds of newcomers flocked to the big tent.

On the next Sunday, and again the following week, Hamblen went on the platform to say, 'I didn't know what it was like to be a real Christian. Do you know the thrill of it all? I like to talk about it. Boy, I talk about it everywhere' – including the bars he had most frequented. He learned that, quite seriously, the betting in 'Gower Gulch' and along Hollywood Boulevard that Hamblen 'wouldn't keep it up', dropped from 100–1 to 20–1; after his second testimony, to 10–1.

The campaign was extended.

At the end of that week Billy, Cliff and Bev Shea put out another 'fleece', praying for a clear sign whether to extend once again.

The night on which they had to make up their minds, Billy arrived at the tent to find the place swarming with reporters and photographers – a new, overwhelming and distracting experience. Flashbulbs exploded everywhere. Billy in the middle of the sermon had to ask a man to climb down from a stepladder he had placed right in front of the platform. All sorts of questions were flung at him afterward, and next day the Los Angeles *Examiner* and *Herald Express* carried banner headlines. The dispatch was featured in the other Hearst papers across the country, and picked up by Associated Press. Someone told Graham, 'You've been kissed by William Randolph Hearst.'

Twenty years later Billy Graham heard what lay behind that 'kiss'.

Among the large staff in the bed-ridden Hearst's Californian home worked a middle-aged maid. Hedla had come in 1947 from Chicago, where she used to hurry home from Moody Church to listen to Songs in the Night. At Los Angeles she went to the 'Canvas Cathedral' during that third week of the Crusade, and next morning, when Hedla was helping the nurse to make Hearst's bed, he questioned her closely. He had given some newspaper support to Youth for Christ and this may have left a vague memory of the name Billy Graham which the Hamblen sensation revived. Hearst listened to the maid's warm account of the services. That afternoon he gave his famous order to 'puff Graham'.

One of those who heard Stuart Hamblen's testimony on the radio was a twice-convicted wire-tapper, Jim Vaus, the prodigal son of a prominent Los Angeles minister. He was driving home after clinching a dangerous deal, but his wife, Alice, knew nothing of his criminal activities.

Vaus was amused, then impressed by Hamblen's words. Next day, on an idle Sunday afternoon drive with Alice, on the spur of the moment Vaus took her to the big tent to 'see what this fellow Graham is like.'

They managed to squeeze on the edge of a bench. Vaus despised the crowd, rated Cliff Barrows and his trombone enthusiastic but amateurish. 'Then Billy Graham stepped to the centre of the platform and I couldn't find anything wrong with him . . . Something about the ease with which he moved, the flash in his eyes, the conviction in his voice, gripped me. His message wasn't new, I had heard it lots of times. What amazed me was there weren't any jokes. It was all Bible. And I knew he was telling the truth.'

45

Billy moved rapidly back and forth on the platform, facing one block of seats, then another; he walked an estimated mile during fifty minutes. Every word of his machine-gun-like delivery was audible throughout the entire tent because he wore, on his tie, a microphone attached to a long cable, controlled by Cliff Barrows. Jim Vaus, as he listened, wrestled with his conscience. The companies he had swindled, the equipment stolen, the money he would make, persuaded him not to believe.

When Graham began the invitation Vaus clenched his fists.

An elderly personal worker with more zeal than tact, gripped his arm and would have been knocked into the sawdust had he not begun praying with bowed head. Vaus heard Billy, who had no idea of his existence, say: 'There's a man in this audience who has heard this story many times before, and who knows this is the decision he should make. Yet again he's saying "No" to God. He is hardening his heart, stiffening his neck, and he's going out of this place without Christ. And yet this may be the last opportunity God will give him to decide for Christ.'

Vaus fought in his mind.

Graham said again, far away up at the platform, his voice coming clear through the amplifiers: 'The only time a man can decide for Christ is when the Holy Spirit of God has brought conviction to his heart. If God is bringing conviction to your heart you dare not say "No". This is your moment of decision.'

Jim Vaus muttered, 'I'll go.'

In the smaller tent he was oblivious of his counsellor, of the others around, of Alice kneeling beside him making her own commitment. Vaus himself was 'busy talking to God . . . I prayed: "Lord, I believe; this time from the bottom of my heart . . . It's going to be almost impossible to straighten out this bewildered, tangled life of mine. But if You'll straighten it out, I'll turn it over to You, all of it."'

As the Vauses left the tent a news photographer ran up. Vaus' first reaction was to flee publicity, the second that it was the best way to make known his break with crime.

'WIRETAPPER VAUS HITS SAWDUST TRAIL.'

The news flashed throughout America, by radio, hitherto impervious to religious revivals, and newsprint. Soon both *Time* and *Newsweek* featured 'the new evangelist', and when Louis Zamperini, Olympic runner and war hero, was converted, the headlines screamed again.

The campaign was now the topic of all Los Angeles, and the crowds pressed to the big tent in such numbers that despite enlargement it could not contain them. On the seventh Sunday it was full at midday for a 2.30 pm service and the street blocked by those unable to get in.

In the final week alcoholics and prostitutes and broken bits of humanity, too shy to enter the tent, would ask for personal workers. Before each service church people stood shoulder to shoulder on every inch of the prayer tent, the leader's desk piled so high with written requests that many could not be mentioned.

The atmosphere in the big tent had nothing of the supposed emotion of a revivalist meeting. It was like an immense divine service. The people came because Graham preached with authority. He brought world affairs right into the 'canvas cathedral'. He preached in the shadow of international crisis, and he preached straight from the Bible.

He had stopped trying to prove that the Bible was true, and just proclaimed its message. 'I found that I could take a simple outline and put a number of pertinent Scripture quotations under each point, and God would use this mightily to cause men to make full commitment to Christ . . . I found they were desperately hungry to hear what God had to say through His Holy Word.'

The numbers who came forward reached totals of two or three hundred a night – a figure which in those days seemed fantastic. For every person prayed with, ten or twenty had to be addressed in a group because of the lack of workers. For the first time Graham began to hear of divorced couples being reunited in the counselling tent.

None of the three who hit the headlines had easy growth as Christians. Louis Zamperini, a famous Olympic runner who came forward, suffered doubts and despondency during the rebuilding of his life. Vaus had the hardship of

47

restitution. Hamblen was fired from his $1,000-a-week programme because he refused to advertise beer. Every opening then closed, until his friend, actor John Wayne, hearing he had not taken a drink in thirty days, said: 'Tell me truthfully, Stuart, have you wanted one?'

'No, John. It is no secret what God can do.'

When Wayne suggested, 'You ought to write a song about "It is no secret what God can do",' Stuart Hamblen found his new vocation. Jim Vaus and Louis Zamperini both found theirs among delinquent boys, Vaus in New York, Zamperini in California. These three were representative of some 4,000 men, women and children who came forward, and additional hundreds whose decisions for Christ were not recorded.

The campaign extended from three weeks to eight. Graham wrote that in a campaign like this, 'all I can think about is preaching. Morning, noon and night I am thinking about sermons, preparing sermons, and more preaching. I forget the world, my own personal affairs and everything.'

He had quite run out of sermons. When Ruth came West again she found him begging outlines from preacher friends, and reading every recommended book he could borrow or buy. 'I remember his desperate straits in Los Angeles, probably the best thing that ever happened to him – this suddenly having to get down and study, especially the Bible. He was thrown back on simple, straight *Biblical* preaching.' He was now exhausted and could not sleep properly, but he had discovered that 'the weaker I become physically, the stronger I become spiritually.'

He set Sunday November 20 as closing day. The big tent, enlarged to 9,000 seats, overflowed. No one could estimate the audience, almost certainly the largest of its kind since Billy Sunday's New York campaign of 1917. And no one could have believed that fourteen years later the turnstiles of the Los Angeles Coliseum would click up 134,254, with 20,000 more outside the gates, to hear Billy Graham on the last night of the Los Angeles Crusade of 1963.

On Monday Ruth and Billy took the train for Minneapolis. The conductor treated them as celebrities. At

48

Kansas City reporters boarded the train, at Minneapolis several prominent clergy joined with Northwestern faculty and the local press to provide a hero's welcome. The Grahams at last realized that Billy had been catapulted into fame. They were bewildered, frightened lest they fail their Lord in these new opportunities, uncertain whether this were a climax or a beginning, yet tremendously encouraged.

'I feel so undeserving of all the Spirit has done,' wrote Billy, 'because the work has been God's and not man's. I want no credit or glory. I want the Lord Jesus to have it all.'

6

An Hour of Decision

Cliff Barrows wrote to a friend on 13 January 1950, from Boston, Massachusetts: 'It is our firm conviction that New England is in the midst of a great awakening, and revival fires seem to be spreading not only throughout the city but in many other sections across this area.'

Three years earlier Billy Graham had agreed to bring his Team for New Year meetings at Boston. Predominantly Roman Catholic, with large minorities of Unitarians and Christian Scientists; reserved, proud and confident of its intellectual supremacy, no city in America might more surely snuff the fire lit at Los Angeles. Instead, the meetings spilled out from Mechanics Hall and historic Park Street church to Boston Garden, the city's largest indoor arena, where on Monday 16 January 16,000 squeezed in, leaving so many outside that Billy had to deliver an unscheduled address from the steps. Newspapermen said Franklin D. Roosevelt himself had never drawn such numbers in Boston. That night, with Ruth beside him, Billy 'felt as great a power in preaching as any other time in my ministry up till then. And when the appeal was given, more than a thousand people responded to receive Christ.'

It was all unbelievable, yet wonderful because spontaneous: no counsellor training, no careful buildup, no advertising except for New Year's Eve. The Team promised to return in the spring. After the service the Grahams took a train for Canada, for a speaking engagement in Toronto. Speeding west across Massachusetts Billy felt a compulsion to get off at Worcester and again at Springfield, to telephone Boston that he would stay in New England. Again and again the feeling came to him that now was the hour. Invitations had poured in; from universities, schools, cities. Any town of New England would book its

50

largest hall to hear Billy Graham. The press would carry his words across the nation. If the Team stayed in New England six months, he felt, God might light a fire in America that never would be put out.

Graham was used to acting on impulse. But he was desperately tired, and he was frightened of the press. 'Whatever I said was being quoted. I didn't have the experience to say the right things. And I was afraid that I was going to say something that would bring disrepute on the name of Christ.' At Niagara Falls where they stayed a day and a night, Billy again 'felt tremendously impelled to call back to Boston and say we would continue.' He let it pass, and afterwards believed that 'unwittingly I disobeyed the voice of God.'

Yet to return would have meant abandoning a long-prepared campaign in Columbia, South Carolina.

And the three weeks in Columbia, first in an auditorium, then in a hurriedly built 'wooden cathedral', and finally in the Carolina stadium, showed that Los Angeles and Boston were only a beginning. As he waited to preach at that closing rally in the stadium on 12 March 1950, with the governor and several distinguished men in the audience, Billy felt the quiet expectancy, and 'a deep longing and hunger on the part of thousands for a personal encounter with God.'

Columbia brought into the Team the veteran Willis Haymaker, who had set up campaigns for many evangelists between the wars. He taught the Graham Team the basic facts of organization. He had a gift for making local leaders prepare together, and above all he emphasized prayer as the secret of revival, getting thousands to pray. He introduced also the word 'Crusade' to describe Billy Graham's evangelism, pointing out that a crusade was not confined to the actual meetings: it included preparation and follow up: 'a crusade goes on and on.' Billy was soon speaking of 'our crusade to bring America to her knees in repentance of sin and faith toward God.'

After Columbia in the South the Team whirled through twenty New England towns from Rhode Island to Maine. A corps of national pressmen had attached itself. At nearly every place Billy had to deliver a second talk to the overflow crowd in the street, often in the rain, and at Houlton, Maine, on the Canadian border the only auditorium large enough was the airport hangar. At one place Billy was close to abandoning the tour through exhaustion. Alone in a hotel room he kneeled on the floor in prayer, and before he finished he could feel strength returning to his body.

The climax came with four nights in the Boston Garden arena and a great open air rally on Boston Common on Sunday April 23. The day before the rally Billy wanted to pray where he would preach, and he strolled up Monument Hill, where the platform was still being constructed, with several friends. One of these friends was John Bolten, a German-born industrialist who had rededicated his life to Christ during the January meetings.

As they prayed, John Bolten had such inward conviction that afterward he took Billy for a walk alone. 'Billy,' he said, 'I believe God's telling me you are going to preach in the great stadiums of every capital city of the world the Gospel of our crucified Lord. I believe the world is ripe and ready to listen.'

One morning the following summer, while attending a conference at Ocean City, New Jersey, Billy and Cliff drove over the bridge across the bay to play golf.

That same morning a Philadelphia clergyman, Dr Theodore Elsner, happened to wake up late at the family summer cottage in Ocean City which he and his son-in-law Fred Dienert, a Philadelphia advertising agent, had rented. Elsner was president of the National Religious Broadcasters. As Elsner shaved he prayed for Billy Graham, who he knew was nearby. As he prayed, a definite sense came to him that Billy Graham was the man to fill the gap left by the recent death of Walter A. Maier, the famous weekly radio preacher who had had the ear of America. Maier had preached a clear evangelical Gospel in the context of the social, political and moral state of the nation.

At noon Elsner drove off to find a lunch counter. He felt a strong impression that he should cross the bridge, although he could easily get a sandwich in Ocean City. On the mainland at Somers Point he saw a roadside diner and walked in. There sat Graham, Barrows and a third golfer, Phil Palermo. Elsner ordered a sandwich but barely touched it for exhorting Billy, until Billy in enthusiasm began to pace up and down the diner. 'How am I going to get on radio?' he asked. 'Who's going to help me?'

Elsner told him of his son-in-law, Fred Dienert, whose senior partner, Walter F. Bennett of Chicago, had handled many religious programmes.

On reflection, Billy rejected the idea; a national weekly programme could be almost a full-time occupation. When next month, at a conference in northern Michigan, two well-dressed strangers introduced themselves as Walter Bennett and Fred Dienert of the Walter Bennett Advertising Company, Billy charmingly sent them away. They reappeared at Montreat, and told him that a peak Sunday afternoon time would shortly be available coast-to-coast on the American Broadcasting Company's network, for an initial thirteen week contract at a total of $92,000, a sum which to Graham appeared astronomical.

Shortly afterward Graham began a six weeks' crusade at Portland, Oregon, where a huge, wooden temporary auditorium had been specially erected. Bennett and Dienert pursued him by telephone and telegram to explain that the programme cost about $7,000 a week; if he raised $25,000 he could go on the air, for after three weeks the gifts of listeners would certainly maintain it. None of his staff had ever seen Billy Graham lose his temper, but he now became irritated with these most persistent partners and refused to see them when they came to Portland. Ten days later they were back again. He used the rear elevator and even the fire escape to avoid them in the hotel lobby. They waited a week, received an appointment at last, only to find that Billy had escaped to Mount Hood for his rest-day, a Monday.

On Tuesday morning at Mount Hood Billy and Grady were breakfasting when a call came from Texas, from Howard Butt, a friend of their own age, heir to the grocery chain. Butt said that if it were true Billy might go on radio, he and their mutual friend, Bill Mead, head of a

53

bakery business, wanted to give $1,000 each to start a fund.

When Billy returned with Grady to the Multnomah Hotel at Portland on Tuesday afternoon, he avoided Bennett and Dienert and retired for his usual rest. Grady walked in with a message that the partners had booked a flight home that evening.

Billy told Grady to send for them.

Bennett and Dienert found him pacing back and forth, dressed in his pyjamas and the golf cap he always wore to keep his hair straight when he rested. He told them he was undecided, but reported the offer of $2,000 and supposed he might contact other wealthy men if only his time permitted.

'Billy,' said Fred Dienert, 'I don't think the money is going to come from a lot of big people.' Bennett and Dienert suggested telling the Portland audience about the opportunity.

At length Billy said, 'Boys, let's pray.'

He knelt by a chair. Walter and Fred lowered themselves to the bedside, and 'Billy really poured out his heart to God.' They had never heard a prayer of such childlike directness.

'Lord, You know I'm doing all that I can,' is Fred Dienert's memory of the words of Billy's prayer. 'You know I don't have any money, but I believe we ought to do this. You know, Lord, I'll put another mortgage on; I'll take the little I have and put another mortgage on.

'Lord, I don't know where the money is, and if I did know where it is, I'm too busy to go out and get it.

'I feel the burden for it, but it's up to You, and if You want this, I want You to give me a sign. And I'm going to put out a fleece. And the fleece is for the $25,000 by *midnight*.'

Walter and Fred stole away. In the taxi to the airport they agreed, in awe, 'You could feel the Presence of God there. You could feel a state of expectancy. God was listening to Billy. Something is going to happen.' At the airport, therefore, they turned around and drove to the crusade, seating themselves unrecognized at the back. A huge crowd had come, which they appraised with satisfaction at about

54

20,000; when the plates were passed the amount ought to be raised.

The moment came for the offering toward crusade expenses; Billy said not a word about radio.

The offering taken, Billy spoke of the radio opportunity. He said he felt he should take this available time for God rather than let it go to a tobacco company or suchlike; that he had no money nor the time to raise it. 'But if any of you folks would like to have a part, I'll be in the office back here at the close of the service tonight.' When he mentioned $25,000, which was a lot of money in 1950, Billy heard a ripple or two of laughter.

Bob Pierce, founder of World Vision and fresh from the Korean battlefront, gave the address that night, reporting at length. Billy followed with the basic points of the Gospel, gave the invitation and then said: 'Shall we pray. Every head bowed, every eye closed . . . You come, as everybody in this place prays for you. You come . . . you hundreds of you come . . . .'

People had far to move from the ends of the building and the overflow seats outside. The time passed slowly. Billy stood at the podium, saying a word or two at intervals. Pierce then rose to address the hundreds who had come forward. Walter looked at Fred. Neither thought many of the audience would wait to see Billy at such a late hour. Fred murmured, 'But God is faithful. Whatever He starts, He finishes.'

At last the audience was released. A long queue soon formed near the back office, where Grady held an old shoe box. Scribbled pledges and dollar notes were thrust in. A lumberman from Idaho left a $2,500 pledge. A couple of youths asking, 'Dr Graham, is chicken feed acceptable?' threw in a handful of change and a dollar, and Billy said, 'God bless you. Thank you.' An old lady in a worn black dress produced a $5 bill. A businessman said he had been one of Dr Maier's most ardent supporters, that Graham should certainly pick up Maier's torch. The man pledged $1,000, with the promise of more.

Grady gave the box to the crusade chairman, Frank Phillips, and the Team went to their favourite eating place, where Bennett and Dienert joined them. Frank Phillips entered excitedly saying that the tally, including the promised $2,000 from Texas, was just $23,500.

They all looked at Billy. 'It's a miracle. You're as good as on the air!' Billy, almost in tears at the generosity and trust of the people, firmly said, No; the fleece was for $25,000 before midnight, $25,000 it must be. The devil might have sent the lesser sum to tempt him. When the two partners offered the balance, Billy refused them.

A subdued Team returned to the hotel shortly before midnight. Billy went to his room, Grady to the mail desk, where he was given three envelopes delivered by hand.

In each was a pledge from somebody unable to wait in the queue: one for $1,000, two for $250. Together they made up the $25,000.

Grady Wilson kept the shoe box in his shirt drawer overnight. Next morning he was told by the bank that if, however briefly, he entered cash and cheques under his name he would be liable for income tax, nor could it go tax-free under 'Billy Graham Radio Fund' unless this were a properly constituted body. He put the money temporarily into the account of the Portland crusade, and Billy called George Wilson, business manager of Northwestern Schools, at Minneapolis.

Wilson flew West, bringing articles of incorporation which he had had drawn up the previous year against some such eventuality, and Billy, Ruth, Cliff and the two unrelated Wilsons signed them to form the Billy Graham Evangelistic Association. The others firmly overrode Billy's strong opposition to the trumpeting of his name. The name would identify, and the name was trusted.

As for a title of the radio programme, Ruth vetoed 'The Billy Graham Hour'. She saw that whereas the name of Billy Graham would rightly endorse the Association, it would be 'the height of poor taste' on a programme primarily designed for millions without definite faith in Christ, to whom it might imply the building of a personal following for a preacher. It was she who suggested *Hour of Decision*.

Meanwhile, unknown to the Grahams, Bennett had

arrived at the American Broadcasting Company's Chicago office to sign the contract on Friday afternoon, only to be told that the New York headquarters had changed their minds and would not sell time to Billy Graham. The decision was final.

Bennett and Dienert flew to New York that night. Although ABC's executive offices were always empty on a Saturday morning, a vice-president entered unexpectedly. He had missed the board meeting but had learned of it by memorandum. 'After a lengthy discussion he agreed that we were entitled to a review. He even contacted one of the top executives on the golf course to set up a meeting for Monday morning. The network deliberated for two days and on Wednesday announced the programme's acceptance.'

At Minneapolis George Wilson set up a one-room office on Harmon Place, a few yards across Loring Park from North Western, and hired one secretary; that seemed enough, for they might not get many gifts or spiritual inquiries.

Billy's friends urged him to speak quietly and slowly on radio, in contrast to his preaching. He rejected the advice. In a careful study of newscasters, commentators and radio preachers he detected that those who spoke fast won the largest audience; he modelled himself on Walter Winchell and Drew Pearson, both subsequently his personal friends. He would cover as much ground as he could, touching social and international issues, packing in illustrations and Bible quotations, each message to be 'straight evangelism calculated to stir the Christian and win the person outside the church to Christ . . . Fast, hard-hitting.'

The *Hour of Decision* (a half hour of time, the word 'Hour' in the title following the normal custom of American radio) went out over 150 stations on ABC network on Sunday November 5, 1950, from Georgia, where Willis Haymaker had set up the Atlanta crusade in a specially constructed tabernacle on the baseball field of the Atlanta Crackers at Ponce de Leon Park. Cliff Barrows introduced and led the crusade choir and audience. Grady Wilson gave a Scripture reading. Bev Shea sang.

Then Billy Graham stepped to the microphone. Three days previously the Chinese had massively intervened in the Korean War and were about to inflict a heavy defeat on United Nations forces. In a wide ranging address Billy emphasized the urgency of the hour and pleaded for a nationwide movement of prayer: 'Faith, more than fighting, can change the course of events today. United, believing, self-humbling, God-exalting prayer now can change the course of history.'

Only at the close did he sound a direct evangelistic call, ending: 'A crucified and a risen Christ will forgive sins, lift burdens, solve problems and give assurance of salvation to many. This experience can be yours, whoever you are, and whatever your circumstances may be, if by faith you will open your heart to Jesus Christ. Right now you can say an eternal "Yes" to Christ, and you can become a partaker of eternal life.'

The programme caught on rapidly. Soon it had earned the highest audience rating ever accorded a religious programme. In eighteen months it was rated higher than most news commentators in daytime Sunday listening.

It made Graham's voice familiar across America and many countries overseas. But an attempt to use the new medium of television was short lived, and it was a few years before Billy broke into television in a different way, greatly widening his ministry.

The *Hour of Decision* had a considerable influence on his development as a preacher. Whereas each crusade or rally brought a different audience and sermon material could be used over and over again, the *Hour of Decision* demanded every week a fresh address of highest calibre, which disciplined him all the more to study the Bible and theology, and to observe and assess contemporary events. And the necessary founding of the Billy Graham Evangelistic Association enabled him to cut away from the traditional 'love offering'. Graham and the Team became salaried members of BGEA. Henceforth, wherever they served, they gave their services free.

7

Harringay 1954

In the last week of February 1954 Billy Graham was crossing the Atlantic in the liner *United States* to his strongest challenge yet: the Greater London crusade.

At the age of thirty-five he could look back on a meteoric rise. He had become the best known preacher in America, and by using outdoor stadiums his crusades, with their blend of warmth and reverence, had reached out to thousands reluctant to attend churches or indoor halls. He had faced the problem of follow up. Billy had brought in Dawson Trotman, founder of the Navigators. Under Trotman's guidance the Team had begun to develop the process which integrated into the local churches an increasing proportion of those who came forward.

Quick to seize opportunities and to recruit experts, Billy had made feature films of crusades and with *Mr Texas*, based on the story of a convert at the Fort Worth, Texas crusade, he had pioneered the use of drama blended to factual reporting as a means of film evangelism. He had become a widely read writer – through a weekly syndicated column, *My Answer*, and by his first best seller, *Peace With God*, a book which would remain a classic, in use all over the world. Down the years Billy would hear again and again from men and women brought to Christ through reading it.

The Washington DC crusade in February 1952 had made Billy Graham well known to political leaders. He became a personal friend of two future Presidents, and of President Eisenhower. He had also paid a pastoral visit to the front line troops during the Korean War.

There had been opposition and many pitfalls, but even allowing for the hand of Providence, it is a wonder more mistakes or misjudgements had not occurred. The Team were preserved by their sincerity and integrity; by humility and their devotional roots, and their grasp of the basic truths of the faith. A happy home life and the influence of Ruth were important; another factor was Graham's sense of humour; another his thirst for knowledge, which made him sure the other man knew more than he. Billy would pick any brain, read any book, explore any situation.

Even more important was a continuing sense of inadequacy: 'The Lord has always arranged my life,' he once said, 'that I have had to keep dependent on Him. Over and over again I went to my knees and asked the Spirit of Wisdom for guidance and direction. There were times when I was tempted to flee from problems and pressures and my inability to cope with them; but somehow, even in moments of confusion and indecision, it seemed I could trace the steady hand of God's sovereignty leading me on.'

And now, approaching England for the best prepared of all crusades to date, he was about to need in full measure his dependence on divine wisdom and his trust in the sovereignty of God.

On Monday, February 22, one day short of Southampton, the first steward of the *United States* tapped on the Grahams' door and handed in a radio news sheet. Billy was stunned to read, date-lined London: 'A Labour Member of Parliament announced today that he would challenge in the Commons the admission of Billy Graham to England on the grounds that the American evangelist was interfering in British politics under the guise of religion.' The Grahams were mystified until the London crusade director, Jerry Beaven, came through on the radio telephone.

It appeared that Hannen Swaffer, a columnist on the left-wing *Daily Herald*, had discovered a prayer calendar prepared in Minneapolis. In a descriptive piece under a picture of London appeared the sentence: 'What Hitler's bombs could not do, socialism with its accompanying evils shortly accomplished.' Deftly touching up the small letter *s* to a capital, Hannen Swaffer under a headline, 'Apologize – or stay away!' had written a blistering article pillorying

Billy Graham as a political adventurer in disguise, who had 'more gravely libelled us than anyone has dared to do since the war,' by attacking the former Socialist (Labour) government. Taking their cue from Swaffer's 'disclosure' the London press was in uproar, hot for Billy Graham's scalp.

The piece had been taken unwittingly from an uncorrected proof of a brochure for American donors. On English advice the word 'socialism' had been corrected, before the brochure's publication, to 'secularism'; the two words were synonymous to Americans and no political reference had been intended. Graham did not even recall the details of the brochure and had never seen the calendar.

Beavan sent an explanation to the press; Graham, and George Wilson in Minneapolis wired apologies to the Member of Parliament, but Swaffer, a Spiritualist, followed up with an attack on 'the wild fanaticism of Billy Graham's evangelism.'

Momentarily, Billy was engulfed by certainty that all was over, and by the injustice of the accusations. Then, swiftly and instinctively he turned to the Bible. Opposition was inevitable; Christ must triumph. When they reached Le Havre it was no effort to send by the *Daily Herald*'s reporter a friendly greeting to Hannen Swaffer.

Coming up Southampton Water the ship was boarded by a tugful of pressmen and photographers. They ignored a film star to crowd round the Grahams, who realized later that the 'socialism' furore had been a blessing in disguise by making Billy front-page news. The reporters were hostile. One even asked Ruth: 'Is it true your husband carries around his own special jug of water for baptism?' After a TV interview on the dockside the Grahams entered customs. When the customs officer said, 'Welcome to England and good luck, Sir. We need you,' Billy was eternally grateful for the encouragement, swiftly followed by a dockworker's 'God bless you, sir. I'm praying for you.'

At Waterloo the Grahams stepped into a sea of happy singing people. Londoners had converged on the terminus until platform ticket machines gave out, post-office vans and taxis were held up, and a harassed official exclaimed, 'If

61

these are Christians it's time we let out the lions!' It was the greatest crowd at Waterloo since the arrival of Mary Pickford and Douglas Fairbanks in 1924. The Grahams left the station to the sound of two thousand voices singing Wesley's hymn, 'And can it be that I should gain/An interest in the Saviour's blood?'

On the day before the crusade was to begin, *The People* newspaper hurled abuse at 'Silly Billy . . . Being bulldozed into loving God by ecstatic young men who talk about him with easy familiarity is something which makes the biggest British sinner shudder.' The atmosphere at the press conference was of cynicism mixed with derision. Hugh Gough, suffragan Bishop of Barking and the only Anglican leader to support, said: 'Well, Billy. If you are to be a fool for Christ's sake, I'll be a fool with you.'

The opening day, Monday, March 1, broke cold and cheerless. Billy spent most of it preparing and at prayer in his hotel. The weather worsened. Billy, his nerves taut, developed a splitting headache. Two American Senators, whose intention to attend the crusade had been announced, cried off, murmuring something about political implications. Billy believed that the American Ambassador, who had washed his hands of him at the 'socialism' dispute, had urged them to stay away. Billy 'had a terrible sinking feeling. I dropped immediately to my knees in prayer and committed the entire matter to the Lord.'

Before the Grahams drove out to Harringay arena in North London a garbled telephone message convinced them that it was barely a quarter full. On their arrival, the forecourt was empty. They could, however, see crowds streaming toward the greyhound stadium beyond. Billy said to Ruth, 'Let's go face it and believe that God has a purpose in it.'

Willis Haymaker came toward the car. 'The arena is jammed! It is full and running over, and thousands are on the other side!' Billy, a little dazed, walked through the door to his special room, to a great sound of hymns from the arena. There stood two smiling Senators, saying 'Billy, we just couldn't let you down!' They had hurried from the Prime Minister and would shortly leave for a formal dinner, but were determined to speak on Billy's behalf.

Squads of pressmen and roving photographers did not make for an atmosphere of worship. (The London dailies had sent an extraordinary array, including theatre and literary critics, foreign and industrial correspondents.) From the moment the choir burst into a verse of 'Blessed assurance, Jesus is mine', followed by the stately cadences of the opening hymn, 'Praise to the Lord, the Almighty', the service had a genuineness and reverence which puzzled the press, still attempting to relate Graham to 'snake-handling fundamentalists' and hysterical demagogues.

He preached on John 3:16: 'God so loved the world, that He gave His only begotten Son, that whosoever believeth in Him should not perish, but have everlasting life.' With his microphone looking like an oversize tie pin he darted back and forth. For English ears on that first evening he talked too fast and seemed inclined to shout, so that his voice became expressionless and less effective, but its impact remained unspoiled. 'I believe there is a worldwide hunger for God. I believe this great crowd is evidence of that hunger for God in London, and,' he went on, daringly as it seemed to his audience, 'before three months have passed I believe we are going to see a mighty revival in London and throughout Great Britain.'

At the last moment before preaching, Billy had hesitated whether to give an invitation on this first, press-distracted night. Bishop Gough said, 'Give it.' To the surprise and gratitude of the London executive, 178 people, 'mostly young but scarcely to be described as of one distinct type,' moved quietly forward, some of them weeping.

Numbers were slightly down the second night, a blend of snow flurries and rain. After that, there was never an empty place throughout three months, despite rearrangement to accommodate more than 12,000. On the first Saturday afternoon Harringay was filling so fast for the evening service that Billy took an unannounced meeting in the arena for the first 5,000, who then left. 'Full up' notices in the tube stations did not stop Londoners pouring toward Harringay. They would not disperse. At 9.15 the arena was emptied again and Billy preached a third sermon. The

63

counselling room had already been enlarged three times, for London's first week was bringing forward inquirers in numbers that America had produced only at the last.

The influence of the crusade, from the beginning, was extraordinary. A change of atmosphere could be felt not only in London but across the country. Suddenly it became easy to talk about religion. Billy Graham was the topic in homes, as in factories, clubs and public houses, giving tongue-tied Christians the opportunity of their lives.

From the first night, too, came the singing in the tube. 'From the seemingly endless queues waiting at the station for tickets one hears wave after wave of song rolling back toward the street,' ran a letter in the *Daily Telegraph*. 'The tube trains are packed with these singing multitudes, and there is a smile on every face. This quite spontaneous demonstration of Christian joy is most impressive, and one cannot fail to observe the effect it has on the passengers who board the trains at subsequent stations.'

They sang the great hymns of the Church. They sang 'Blessed Assurance' with its chorus, which Cliff had made the signature tune of the crusade. One song caught on right across London: 'To God be the glory, great things He hath done.' Words and tune are nineteenth-century American yet until London they had not been known to the Team, who now adopted the hymn as their own for its apt expression of their message, experience and aim.

By the third week of March opposition had melted. The press had turned from vociferous suspicion to a respect which soon became admiration and support.

From London and all southern England the crowds flocked to Harringay, from curiosity, conviction, or by invitation of churches or friends. Many came because of the change in others. When a typist saw a colleague suddenly stop being disgruntled, when a store manager was handed back stolen goods by a contrite customer, they wanted to know why.

A large percentage of those who came forward were between the ages of fifteen and twenty-five, the younger ones often being members of church youth groups whose leaders had prayed and worked for their decisions. In older age groups many had an early, lost background of religion. Decision cards showed more than half of no regular church connection. In every Harringay audience many had never been to a religious service other than a wedding or a funeral; or they were like the pickpocket who said to the stranger beside him as they started for the front, 'Now I must give you back your wallet I took a few minutes ago!'

Malcolm Muggeridge, not then a Christian, commented on BBC television: 'One or two at first, and then the movement gathering momentum, as the choir sings quietly. I looked at their faces, so varied, so serious, and for me this was far and away the most moving part of the proceedings.' As the weeks wore on, Billy Graham put less and less force into the invitation. 'I felt,' he said, 'like a spectator standing on the side watching God at work, and I wanted to get out of it as much as I could and let Him take over.'

On Monday, March 29, the Greater London crusade extended itself nationwide.

The American Broadcasting Company's engineer travelling with the Team to supervise *Hour of Decision* broadcasts, hit on the idea of hiring long-distant telephone lines. The BBC used them, and long ago a speech by Lloyd George had been relayed from a hall in London to a hall in the provinces. After some hesitation the post office offered terms.

The first relay was laid to a cinema just across the Thames; the next night 2,000 people in Glasgow heard Billy Graham in London; soon the post office had more applications than they could manage. The services were often clearer to a relay audience than in the arena with its echoing amplifiers, and the message came in stark simplicity unaided by atmosphere or the personality of the preacher. In hired theatres, concert halls, city auditoriums and churches, Britons heard Billy Graham.

In London the crusade went from strength to strength. On Saturday afternoon, April 3, Trafalgar Square was packed as it had not been since VE day. On Good Friday, April 16, sunny and warm, an open-air rally in Hyde Park, at which the police estimated there were more than 40,000, covered half a square mile. Graham spoke with great power on 'God forbid that I should glory, save in the cross of our Lord Jesus Christ.'

Holy Week had been designated a rest period without meetings, but the Team sensed that it would be an error to break the momentum. Even Sundays were filled. On April 25 Billy preached at Cambridge in the packed University Church, with the service relayed in two neighbouring churches. On another Sunday he preached in Birmingham at the annual service of the British Industries Fair. Almost every day he met leading men in church and state, individually or in groups.

The strain was immense. Each week Billy looked thinner, and the rings under his eyes blacker. A distinguished physician prescribed vitamin pills; they had such big effect and looked so small that Billy, prescribed one a day, took four!

If London exhausted him physically (and a man much over thirty-five could scarcely have stood the strain), the Greater London crusade gave Billy Graham new stature.

America had followed his troubles and read of his triumphs with such avid interest that he now became a household name to his countrymen. And Harringay lastingly influenced his ministry. He learned to speak more slowly and quietly; in dress, he abandoned the loud ties which had suggested superficial showmanship. Similarly, Cliff Barrows stopped using his trombone to stir the singing. All of the Team were steadied and matured by working with British Christians, and were encouraged to find themselves reaching not only a capital but a nation.

The crusade already had drawn a million and a half and had been extended again and again until it was announced that the closing service, on the evening of Saturday, May 22, would be held in London's largest outdoor stadium, Wembley, where the soccer league's Cup Final is played. The bookings became so heavy that the smaller White City stadium, a few miles south, was taken for an additional service the same afternoon (even that was not enough; an overflow crowd had to listen in a neighbouring football ground.)

The last day of the Greater London crusade, May 22,

1954, brought weather as unpropitious as the first. Nothing else was the same for Billy as he awoke, weary. The previous evening Harringay had filled so early that two and a half hours before the service the BBC broadcast police warnings that without a ticket one should stay home. And the morning news was of special trains and coaches converging on London, and of people camping out, despite the cold and wet, to make sure of places at White City or Wembley, where the Lord Mayor would be present and the Archbishop of Canterbury, Geoffrey Fisher, once so cautious and negative about Graham, would give the benediction.

After Graham's sermon at White City some 2,000 inquirers walked out of the stands and crossed the running track toward the platform, to stand in the drizzle. The police said the roads round Wembley were chaotic with traffic. Too late to hire a helicopter the Team moved across by a bus under police escort, to reach Wembley in time for tea with the Archbishop, Lord Mayor and the other distinguished guests. As Billy, who 'just did not know where I was going to find the strength for the sermon', looked out of the window, amazed to see every seat in the enormous oval already filled, the gates were opened and an overflow was allowed to swarm onto the precious turf. That cold wet evening witnessed the greatest religious congregation, 120,000 by turnstile count, ever seen until then in the British Isles.

On the platform during the first half hour, which was being broadcast, Billy glanced at the Archbishop and other great men near him and was suddenly tempted to switch from his simple message to 'something impressive in an intellectual framework.' He rejected the temptation and preached again in simplicity, without trace of his weariness, ending: 'You can go back to the shop, the office, the factory, with a greater joy and peace than you have ever known. But before that can happen you must commit yourselves to Jesus Christ. You must make your personal decision for Him. And you can do that now. Choose this day whom ye will serve!'

The *News of the World* described the scene that followed:

'There was no emotional hysteria, no tension . . . only a very deep reverence . . . Within minutes thousands of men, women and teenagers were moving to the track. They were of all ages, of all classes of society. Husbands and wives were hand in hand with their children, young men walked forward alone.' The Archbishop stepped to the microphones and prayed.

Afterwards, as the Team's bus inched slowly through the crowds waving goodbye and singing, 'To God be the glory', Billy stood up. 'I want all of us to bow our heads right now and give thanks to God for all He has done and is doing. This is His doing, and let none fail to give Him credit.'

When Billy had prayed, Bev Shea, the whole Team joining, began to sing softly, 'Praise God from Whom all blessings flow'.

On the day after Wembley, Billy Graham went to Oxford University to address a packed congregation. On the Monday, lying in bed in his London hotel, which he was to leave that night for a holiday in Scotland, he was summoned at short notice to 10 Downing Street by Sir Winston Churchill.

Billy had written inviting the Prime Minister to Wembley. Papers concerning Harringay were placed before Churchill, and he consulted his party's Chief Whip before deciding not to attend. One of his principal private secretaries, Sir John Colville, who had met Billy at a luncheon, asked the Prime Minister if he would see him, but Churchill said, 'No'. However the reports of Wembley so impressed him that Sir Winston agreed to give Graham five minutes, intending merely to be civil. As the hour approached, Sir Winston paced back and forth, saying he was nervous about the encounter: 'What do you talk to an American evangelist about?'

At the stroke of noon Billy Graham was shown into the Cabinet Room. Sir Winston stood at the centre of the long Cabinet table, an unlighted cigar in his hand. Billy was surprised to see how short a man he was. Sir Winston motioned Billy to be seated and said he had been reading about him and was most happy to have him come, 'because we need this emphasis.' Then he said, 'Do you have any hope? What hope do you have for the world?'

Billy was naturally overwhelmed at meeting privately the greatest man of the age, but did not forget why he had been allowed the privilege. He took out his little New Testament and answered, 'Mr Prime Minister, I am filled with hope.'

Sir Winston pointed at the early editions of three London evening papers lying on the empty table, and commented that they were filled with rapes, murders and hate. When he was a boy it was different. If there was a murder it was talked about for fifty years. Everything was so changed now, so noisy and violent. And the Communist menace grew all the time. 'I am an old man,' he said, and repeated the phrase at different points in the conversation nine times. Several times he added, 'without hope for the world.'

Billy said again that he was filled with hope. 'Life is very exciting even if there's a war, because I know what is going to happen in the future.' Then he spoke about Jesus Christ, and began right at the beginning, turning from place to place in the New Testament and explaining, just as he would to an insignificant inquirer in his hotel room, the meaning of Christ's birth, His death, His resurrection and ascension, and how a man is born again. He moved quickly, inwardly agitated lest he should not put across the essentials in the short time granted him.

Billy got the impression that Churchill was very receptive. He made little comment but listened closely – a different attitude from that which Churchill is reported to have shown to ecclesiastical dignitaries. He sat well forward in his chair, drinking in every word.

The five minutes which he had scheduled for Graham had become forty, and the clock showed twelve-thirty, when at last Sir Winston stood up. 'I do not see much hope for the future,' he said, 'unless it is the hope you are talking about, young man. We must have a return to God.'

Harringay had encouraged that return throughout the nation. At the final ministers' meeting in Central Hall, Westminster, the Bishop of Barking said: 'A new flame of hope has been lit in our hearts, new courage and new faith. A fire has been lit which will continue, please God, if we are willing to obey the guidance of God's Holy Spirit in the days and years to come.'

The widespread feeling in the country was nowhere more beautifully expressed than in a private letter written on behalf of Queen Elizabeth the Queen Mother, by her Treasurer, in reply to Billy Graham's invitation to attend the closing service at Wembley[1]:

'I write at the desire of Queen Elizabeth The Queen Mother in reply to your recent letter, to which Her Majesty has given, since she received it in Scotland, a very full and sympathetic consideration.

'Her Majesty bids me tell you of the deep interest with which she has followed the course of your visit to England.

'The immediate response to your addresses, and the increasing number of those who are anxious to hear them, testify both to your own sincerity and to the eagerness with which a great host of the people of this country welcome the opportunity to fortify their religious belief and to reaffirm the principles which you proclaim.

'It is not possible for Queen Elizabeth The Queen Mother to be present on the 22nd, but she wishes me to tell you how impressed she has been by the spiritual rekindling you have brought to numberless Englishmen and women whose faith has been made to glow anew by your addresses.

'Her Majesty would like to pay her tribute both to the manner of your presentation and to its result, and to wish you Godspeed in your task.'

1. Quoted by gracious permission of Her Majesty Queen Elizabeth The Queen Mother.

8

Ripe for Harvest

Sixty thousand stood in the rain and mud when Billy preached on Monday, June 7, 1954 at Cliff College in Derbyshire; outside hotels on his journey people gathered in the streets, hoping to see him; in Glasgow, for discussions with Scottish church leaders, the police had to hold back the crowds.

Graham became alarmed and confused. The expectancy was prodigious. He had invitations to all major cities of Britain. He wondered whether he should abandon his imminent preaching tour in continental Europe, and crusades scheduled in America, and after a rest return to Britain in the late summer for as long as needed.

Weighing on him even more than cancelling crusades was a fear lest 'there was too much interest in me as a person . . . There might be a Billy Graham sect forming, and I might do something to hurt the church in Britain.' He laid his fears before the Archbishop of Canterbury. Dr Fisher advised Graham to wait a year.

With other counsellors divided and plans already forward for 1955, he decided to accept Fisher's advice. Years afterwards, with hindsight, Billy regretted that fatigue had affected his judgement: he should have stayed.

Meanwhile he flew to Scandinavia, Holland and West Germany. So great was the interest generated by London that long-planned one-day meetings were changed to huge stadium rallies. But the night after the rally at Düsseldorf he woke with a wracking, stabbing pain in the small of the back. A specialist diagnosed kidney stone. Against medical advice Billy flew on to Berlin where he was to preach in the Olympic stadium: the Berlin Wall had not yet been built and thousands would cross from the eastern zone. The communist newspapers were attacking him, and Billy could not imagine then that twenty-nine years later he would preach in east Berlin and cities of eastern Germany.

On the morning before the rally the pain returned. Billy refused a stronger pain-killer because it would make him sleepy. He mused to John Bolten, at his bedside: 'Why is God doing this to me? . . . I know what it is. I have just had a wonderful crusade in England. God has blessed me beyond imagination, and now I'm going to preach in Hitler's stadium before 100,000 people. And I would have probably talked to them in my own strength. God is humbling me. He is not going to divide His honour with anybody. He is telling me to lay everything at His feet and ask Him to fill the empty Billy with His own strength.'

They drove in a long motorcade down Hitler's route. Bolten, who had known Hitler personally and had broken with him in 1928, reflected how 'a young Timothy with a very different message now went the same road to the same place.' Instead of Nazi songs the hymns of the Reformation echoed round the stadium. Where the swastika had stood was the text: 'I am the Way, the Truth and the Life.' When Billy preached, none could have told that he was ill.

He preached also in Paris, then sailed home on 1 July, to a hero's welcome in New York harbour. He refused a most lucrative contract for a film on his life and returned to Montreat, where the small house on Assembly Drive received endless telephone calls, an avalanche of mail, and became a focus for inquisite tourists. A good rest seemed impossible – until fresh pains led to removal of the kidney stone, and orders to cancel engagements for six weeks.

That winter of 1954–55, while Billy Graham, Cliff Barrows and Bev Shea held crusades in America, the British Isles were looking forward to the six weeks' All-Scotland Crusade based on Kelvin Hall, Glasgow. For the first time Billy Graham would come with the official endorsement of the churches to lead a united effort to reach an entire land – the land of his ancestors.

The preparations had a vital influence on the Team's development. In previous crusades clergymen had been invited by letter to send likely counsellors to the classes, and perhaps seven or ten would come from each church. At

Glasgow the clergy were nervous about what might be taught. Jerry Beavan and Charlie Riggs therefore explained the training programme to groups of a hundred ministers each from the city and surrounding counties. Many of these sent in fifty or more names: nearly 4,000 persons took the classes. The highest hitherto had been Harringay with 2,500; in America it had been much smaller. Thenceforth the Team always explained follow-up to the clergy first.

A solid cross section of church people began to learn how to be counsellors. To many Scots this use of the Bible was new. Furthermore many were converted in the counselling classes which thus became one of the most important aspects of the crusade.

Billy Graham came to Glasgow on the morning of March 9, 1955, waved to by singing groups as the train from the south rushed through wayside stations, and welcomed at St Enoch Station by an enthusiastic crowd. 'Glasgow Belongs to Billy', ran the headline in a paper that evening.

He had no fear of empty seats the first night of Kelvin Hall. The crusade being intended for all Scotland, the greater part of the space had to be reserved for organized parties; tickets for the whole six weeks were taken before the start, and an annex with closed-circuit TV, holding 3,000, was hurriedly arranged. For unreserved seats people were queuing outside Kelvin Hall throughout the raw afternoon.

Many ministers had questioned whether Billy should invite public decisions. To come forward, rather than to wait behind or file into another room, was most un-Scottish. In reply to the doubts of the chairman, Tom Allan, Billy said, 'Let's see what happens.' Allan could detect in him – and before every subsequent meeting – 'an inner and very finely controlled tension . . . A man under immense strain but somehow living on top of the strain.' Once Billy had prayed with his friends and the meeting began he seemed to Allan transformed: 'All the strain is gone, and from then on the man has forgotten himself.'

The first night, attended by a galaxy of notables, was most unemotional and somewhat chaotic, with coughs, photographers, and constant movement on creaking boards in different parts of the hall. The choir was superb. Bev

Shea, recovering from laryngitis, sang one verse only. During the early part of the service Billy had a moment of lost confidence, perhaps because everybody anticipated a great victory, whereas at Harringay they had half-expected failure. But when he rose there was a great hush. 'I have never felt an audience so close to me before,' Graham wrote to Ruth. 'It seemed that the hearts were open and the Lord pouring it in. I tried to talk quietly and deliberately. I could feel the power of the Holy Spirit moving in the audience.

'Then came the moment of decision. Would they come? Would they respond?

'I asked them to bow their heads, and then quietly gave the invitation. At first not a person moved. My heart began to sink a little. My faith wavered only for a second, and then it all came flooding back to me that millions of people were praying and that God was going to answer their prayers. Then great faith came surging into my heart, and I knew they would come even before I saw the first one move. I bowed my head and began to pray. Then I glanced up and people were streaming from everywhere. I saw some of the ministers with their clerical collars, on the platform, begin to weep.'

The All Scotland Crusade did not have to make its way as at Harringay, but was borne along in a floodtide of goodwill and spiritual hunger.

Every audience was a true cross section of social levels; whereas Harringay had reached directly only a small proportion of artisans and manual workers, in Glasgow almost all parishes co-operated including those mainly of dockers and steel workers.

And the crusade reached the unchurched by a new scheme: Operation Andrew. Introduced to the Team during Harringay, Operation Andrew (named from the incident in the gospels when Andrew brought Simon Peter to Jesus) encouraged churches to charter coaches on which members could only travel if they brought along non-churchgoers. Churches were invited to book reservations at Kelvin Hall according to the spirit of Operation Andrew. 'The idea,' says Riggs, 'was to go out after the uncommitted, the unchurched, and bring them in a group.'

In Glasgow the scheme was experimental and unpolished, but it became a vital factor in the ever-widening influence of the Graham crusades throughout the world.

On Good Friday the service at Kelvin Hall was carried live by television and radio throughout Great Britain.

Graham had approached the occasion somewhat fearfully, for he must preach simultaneously to three audiences, each requiring a different approach: viewers, listeners, and those present in the hall. Determined that nothing should be theologically ill-digested, he took an opportunity to pick the brains of Scotland's foremost theologian, and he was also determined 'to make the gospel so simple that the smallest child might understand.' In his preparation, as he meditated on the cross, he felt 'my unworthiness and sinfulness.'

Good Friday in the Britain of 1955 was still predominantly a religious day. There was only one TV channel, and that night, with his sermon on the Cross, Graham reached more people than any other preacher in Britain before him, including a television audience second only to the Coronation. In public houses rough men sat with eyes glued to the screen in utter quiet; at football matches next day it was the chief topic at half time. The service was watched in Buckingham Palace and in tenement rooms. Not only was it (in the professional opinion of *TV Mirror*) 'unmistakably superb television', but the content was crystal clear, proclaiming Christ's death in man's stead so plainly that the issues, even if rejected, could not be misunderstood.

Throughout the next week Scotland from the Outer Hebrides to the East Coast was linked to Kelvin Hall by a national relay mission. The haphazard landline relays from Harringay were the inspiration for the brilliantly conceived plan of a veteran Scots evangelist of the Church of Scotland, D. P. Thomson, who organized thirty-seven relay centres, each with trained counsellors and its own missioner to take over after Graham's invitation had been heard from Glasgow. The relay mission ended with a rally at Tynecastle Stadium outside Edinburgh. During the final two weeks the services in Kelvin Hall were relayed to many centres in England, Wales and Ireland.

75

The All Scotland crusade ended in glory with two stadium rallies at Glasgow. It had seen a great reaping where others had sown, and created immense expectancy. The next General Assembly of the Church of Scotland gave Billy Graham a thunderous welcome. To the son of staunch Scottish Presbyterians, this was 'one of the most historic moments of my entire ministry.'

After a short holiday the Team went south. Wembley stadium had been taken for a week, a daring innovation: Graham had never yet returned to a city for a second crusade, and no stadium of comparable size had been taken for seven nights.

Every factor weighed against it. The new Prime Minister, Eden, called a general election which absorbed energies and interest. Billy drew greater crowds – 50,000 or 60,000 every night – than any politician, but the London newspapers, recovering from a strike, gave little coverage. The weather was atrocious: every night except two it poured, and those two were bleak. Many who had taken free reservations stayed away to leave empty seats, and though attendance far outpaced Harringay, even the final congregation of 80,000 seemed a contrast to the unforgettable close of 1954.

The rain did not stop inquirers swarming across – in numbers that also dwarfed Harringay – at the close of each service, about 3,000 a night. These gave a fine opportunity to converts of 1954, some 400 of whom were among the counsellors. Many of the organizers, however, were disappointed. Billy Graham himself found Wembley, quite apart from the rain, one of his hardest crusades, for it was his first with an audience so far away as to be almost impersonal.

All adverse factors would have been outweighed had the foremost church leaders identified themselves with this new attempt to reach the unchurched. Archbishop Fisher and many diocesans had written warmly about Harringay but none of them supported Billy at Wembley.

In contrast to the hesitation of high ecclesiastics, the British royal family stretched out hands in friendship.

Billy and Ruth spent forty-five minutes with the Queen Mother and Princess Margaret at Clarence House, and were touched to discover a detailed knowledge of the meetings in London and Scotland and of their family life. Much of the conversation revolved round spiritual matters. The Duchess of Kent (Princess Marina) paid a private visit to the Wembley service. On the Sunday Billy Graham preached before the Queen and the Duke of Edinburgh, the Queen Mother and Princes Margaret, and a small congregation of royal household and estate workers at the Chapel Royal, Windsor Great Park. 'I preached in utter simplicity . . . I had prayed so much that I knew that however simple and full of mistakes my sermon was, God would overrule it and use it.' Afterwards the Grahams had luncheon with the Queen, the first of several luncheons or other private meetings down the years.

The Queen's invitation was a fitting tribute to the fourteen months in 1954–55 in which Billy Graham and his Team had influenced British religion to a marked degree. Churches were revived, many put evangelism into their programmes for the first time. The crusades in London and Glasgow had presented clergy and ministers with a pastoral opportunity unparalleled in the first half of the twentieth century. They gave British Christianity a strong impetus throughout the later 1950s. Too many churches, however, held back, debating the pros and cons instead of recognizing their hour. Had they maintained the momentum, the 1960s might have been as different for Britain nationally, despite the flooding in of secularism, as they were for the thousands who through the crusades of 1954–55 found faith or vocation.

These were the lasting fruit, especially the young. There was a sharp increase in the number of men offering for ordination, and of men and women training for lay or missionary service. By 1959 the Bible Institute in Glasgow had more students than it could house. In 1966, during Billy Graham's next London crusade at Earls Court, the future Bishop of Norwich, Maurice Wood, brought together one night seventy men and women training for full time service as a result of Harringay or Wembley. By the 1980s many converts of these crusades were in positions of leadership or high responsibility, not in Britain only but

77

wherever Britons served the churches: Billy Graham frequently met or learned of such men and women when he held overseas crusades.

The fame of the British crusades led to Graham's first major opportunity away from the West, in January 1956. Invitations had poured in from every part of the world and he had accepted that from India. It had been endorsed by almost every church and mission except Roman Catholic, the first time in India's history that such multiplicity of Christian endeavour had united behind one man, and preparations had been made on a scale never known.

The meetings were of a size unprecedented for a Christian preacher, and public interest was almost as great among Hindus as within the Christian minority. At each place Billy preached basically the same address on the text, John 3:16, and spoke in short sentences for easy interpretation. 'When I gave the invitation,' he wrote to Ruth from Madras, 'all you could hear was just the tramp, tramp, tramp of bare feet and sandalled feet as they were coming forward quietly and reverently . . . I have never seen such sincerity and devoutness on the faces of people. This was God. Yes, the same God that was with us at Wembley and Harringay and Kelvin Hall has been with us here in India.'

India captivated Billy. He warmed to the indefinable sense of exhilaration in the cold weather season. He loved the sights and sounds, the jostling of ancient and modern, the gracefulness of the people, the teeming life of the cities and the placid timelessness of the villages. Its poverty tore at him and he had to be rescued from scattering rupees.

In the last days of January he reached Kerala, the heart of South India's ancient indigenous Christianity. He spoke in Kottayam cathedral to a congregation that included the Jacobite Catholicos of the East in his red robes, bearded Mar Thoma bishops in purple or white, and the famous Bishop Jacob, leader in the formation of the Church of South India.

Billy had been awakened early by the blaring of amplifiers in the specially enlarged college athletic field below the bishop's house. He peeped out and saw a great prayer meeting in progress under arc lights. He preached that night to a concourse which could not be counted, but was believed locally to be far in excess of 75,000. The quiet reverence and intentness, even the silence of food vendors and bookstall keepers during the service, brought home to Billy the strength of Christianity in South India. He saw that the key to the evangelization of India lay among Indians themselves, a conviction by no means universally held by western missionaries in 1956. He resolved to do his utmost to aid Asians to preach Christ to Asians.

He was already doing so. At Madras, as Graham preached, his Tamil interpreter, Victor Monogoram, became so involved in evangelizing, as distinct from merely translating, that his own ministry received new power. At Delhi the interpreter was an outstanding intellectual, Dr Akbar Abdul-Haqq. Haqq had nearly refused to interpret because he had never done such work, but mostly because 'I was not interested in this sort of outreach at all, even though I was curious to find out how God was using Billy Graham.' During the first of the Delhi meetings Billy sensed that his interpreter was 'God's chosen vessel for this type of evangelism in the Orient,' and startled Haqq next day by saying: 'I'm not the man to be used for spiritual awakening here. It has to be an Asian. I think you are the man.'

By the end of that year Akbar Haqq had joined the Billy Graham Team and begun his great ministry of 'Good News Festivals' in India, preaching also at American universities and as an associate in many of Graham's crusades.

Billy Graham capped his Indian tour by one-day rallies in six countries of the Far East, each leading to full crusades later. In India his visit had heartened and stirred the churches and awoken widespread desire for revival and evangelism.

To Billy himself the tour of 1956 brought renewed conviction 'that human nature is the same the world over, and that when the Gospel of Christ is preached in simplicity and power, there is a response in the human soul.'

9

New York 1957

New York with its polyglot population, its fierce competitive spirit, its hustle and sophistication and absorption in things material – a crusade in the city of Wall Street, of Broadway, Madison Avenue and Harlem and all that those names connoted might be a disaster. Protestants were in a minority to Roman Catholics and Jews, church-going in Manhattan was low, and a contemporary expert likened evangelism in New York to 'digging in flint.'

Billy Graham accepted an invitation from the Protestant Council of the City of New York, representing 1,700 churches of 31 denominations, and from a number of independent bodies. All the important churches would co-operate, at least in name, for a six weeks' crusade to begin on May 15, 1957, in the old Madison Square Garden. The committee took an option for a further five months.

During the two years of preparation Billy's acceptance of the invitation brought upon his head some of the most violent opposition he had experienced.

The *Christian Century*, at that time in full tilt against him, derided the coming crusade: 'The Graham procedure ... does its mechanical best to "succeed" whether or not the Holy Spirit is in attendance. At this strange new junction of Madison Avenue and Bible Belt, the Holy Spirit is not overworked; He is overlooked.' Extreme fundamentalists, including some older men who Graham had revered, attacked him for being sponsored by 'modernists', although the crusade was not organized by the Protestant Council (which included many liberals) but by an executive committee of fifteen men who shared Graham's basic outlook and aims. And no one controlled the preaching except Graham, who intended 'to pull no punches in presenting Christ and Him crucified.'

While enduring these attacks Billy Graham met a succession of problems 'far too big for me, that could destroy the crusade', including the death of Dawson Trotman in a boating accident, which meant switching the leadership of counselling and follow up training; and the crusade director's resignation for personal reasons. Charlie Riggs took over. 'I did not think Charlie could do it,' Graham recalls, 'except I had this peace – that Charlie so depended on God and the Holy Spirit that I knew the Lord could do it through Charlie.'

The scale of the preparation looked immense for the times: to provide adequate numbers for each night some 4,000 people were training for the choir, 5,000 took counselling classes, 3,000 volunteered as ushers. And the New York churches were increasingly wholehearted – largely through the work of a comparatively new Team Associate, Billy's young brother-in-law from Canada, Leighton Ford, who won the clergy's confidence to a marked degree. And during the Team's devotional retreat, as the crusade drew near, Leighton Ford gave a 'searching, challenging, convicting message', through which, wrote Graham, 'We were all broken by the Holy Spirit.' By the end of the retreat they felt cleansed and anointed for the task ahead.

When Billy Graham reached New York he felt physically fitter and spiritually better prepared than before any previous crusade, yet 'more inadequate and helpless'. There had been ample predictions that he would fail. 'From human viewpoint and by human evaluation it may be a flop,' Graham commented. 'However, I am convinced in answer to the prayers of millions that in the sight of God and by heaven's evaluation it will be no failure. God will have His way, and in some unknown and remarkable way Christ will receive the glory and honour.'

'We have not come to put on a show or an entertainment. We believe that there are many people here tonight that have hungry hearts – all your life you've been searching for peace and joy, happiness, forgiveness.

'I want to tell you, before you leave Madison Square

Garden this night of May 15, you can find everything that you have been searching for, in Christ. He can bring that inward deepest peace to your soul. He can forgive every sin you've ever committed. And He can give you the assurance that you're ready to meet your God, if you will surrender your will and your heart to Him.

'I want you to listen tonight not only with your ears, but the Bible teaches that your heart also has ears. Listen with your soul tonight. Forget that there's anyone else here. Forget me as the speaker, listen only to the message that God would have you to retain from what is to be said tonight.

'Shall we pray: *Our Father and our God, in Christ's name we commit the next few moments to Thee, and we pray that the speaker shall hide behind the Cross until the people shall see none, save Jesus.*

'*And we pray that many tonight will re-evaluate their relationship to God, others will consider, for the first time perhaps, their need of God, and that many shall respond and surrender themselves to Him as they did 2,000 years ago on the shores of Galilee: for we ask it in His name. Amen.*'

Billy Graham's prayer on that opening night was answered. From the start the crusade made an unprecedented impact on the city of New York and broke all records. The total attendance of more than two million was the highest of any event in the history of Madison Square Garden. More than 60,000 people came forward, swamping the follow-up system until it was reorganized. They were a cross section of society: 'the socially prominent and the outcast, the rich and the poor, the illiterate who could not sign their own decision cards and the university professor; racial lines were freely crossed and Negroes and Puerto Ricans were among the large groups.' A Team associate, Dr Robert O. Ferm, who questioned a large number one year later, wrote that 'the utter fascination of listening to the reports of converts would convince the sceptic that a work of grace had been done. The person who actually made the decision retains a warm and vibrant faith that has been able to survive and persist through many discouragements and above many obstacles.'

The press gave extensive coverage. *The New York Times* printed the entire text of Graham's sermon on several occasions. *The Herald Tribune* allowed him space on the front page to write whenever he wished. There were critical articles too. The great theologian Reinhold Niebuhr in *Life* magazine stated that Graham's evangelism 'neglected to explore the social dimensions of the Gospel.' Neibuhr admitted that Graham 'had sound personal views on racial segregation and other social issues of our time,' but alleged that 'he almost ignores them in his actual preaching.'

Niebuhr based this opinion on the newspaper accounts of the crusade and on occasional attendance. The Associated Press religious writer, George W. Cornell, sitting at the press desk night after night, disagreed with this view. He wrote a private letter to Graham: 'I have read various criticisms of you from those who say you do not stress the full social implications of Christ's demands (the horizontal aspects, as you put it), but I have concluded that the critics simply have not paused to listen to you, but have been so dazzled by your external successes that they don't see its roots.' Nevertheless, Niebuhr's criticism was taken to heart; Graham increasingly touched on a whole range of social issues.

President Mackay of Princeton Theological Seminary wrote: 'Men have been made aware of the sins of the heart and of society. It is unfair to demand that Billy Graham should have offered a blueprint for the solution of complicated social issues in our highly industrialized mass society.' But this was just what his critics did demand, for they rejected his belief that the root ill of human society is the unregenerate human heart.

Ethel Waters, celebrated black singer and actress, made a spontaneous retort on television to the question whether the crusade would fail: 'God don't sponsor no flops!'

Her remark was heard by Lane Adams, the former fighter pilot and night club singer who had postponed ordination to direct the crusade's outreach to show business people. He offered her a seat in the reserved section. During her long stage and screen career Ethel Waters had never lost the consciousness of God that had come when she was converted at the age of twelve, and as she walked into Madison Square Garden that first night she 'felt that my Lord was calling me back home.'

After the first week she joined the choir of fifteen hundred voices in order to secure a reserved seat every night, and sang at each service for eight weeks. 'So many things I had pondered about for a lifetime, the Lord cleared up during these weeks.' Cliff Barrows learned of her presence when she signed a choir petition for the extension of the crusade, and asked her if she would sing a solo. She sang the song that she made famous on Broadway: 'His Eye is on the Sparrow'. 'This time, however, it was to be very different. The glitter and heartache of the stage had disappeared . . . There was just myself, standing before 18,000 people, saying, "I love Jesus, too," the only way I could say it – by singing "His Eye is on the Sparrow".'

On five nights in the final eight weeks Ethel Waters sang that song. When the crusade ended she had readjusted much in her life, for 'I found that I could no longer act every role I was offered and continue to glorify my Lord.' She played in the feature film based on the New York crusade, *The Heart is a Rebel*, and visited crusades year by year, at her own expense, to sing in her inimitable style, until her death in 1977.

The coming of Ethel Waters, who in her own way became virtually a member of the Team, was one of the crusade's long term effects on the Billy Graham story. But by far the most significant was the breakthrough into television.

It was not premeditated. A few days after the crusade began Fred Dienert said to Billy Graham: 'Wouldn't it be wonderful if we could take this crowd to the nation, if the people at home could see what's going on, and the people coming to Christ.' Graham, recalling the great influence on Britain of the Kelvin Hall telecast on Good Friday 1955, agreed. Bennett and Dienert sounded the networks about televising the crusade coast-to-coast, but encountered scepticism, even ridicule. Then the American Broadcasting

Company offered time, and a foundation offered the money to pay for the first four hour-long telecasts.

These telecasts on Saturday June 1 and each following Saturday (seventeen in all) from the country's best known arena were a revelation to America. As a television ministry it was a thousand times more effective than the Graham Team's studio programme of earlier years, for the crowd in the Garden created a strong sense of participation for the viewer, who was now eavesdropping an event, not watching a contrived half hour of song and talk.

After the first telecast over 25,000 letters came in, to encourage or thank Billy Graham, or to tell of decisions made for Christ while viewing. Each succeeding Saturday widened and deepened the influence of the television crusade. In Chicago, at Polk Brothers' display of TV sets at the Chicagoland Fair, so many people watched those sets that happened to be tuned in to the crusade, and ignored the others, that the sales representatives went down the long line and turned all sets to the crusade. In Buffalo the Council of Churches reported that criticism of the New York crusade had been swept away and that church attendance had reached an unprecedented figure for the time of year.

The first television crusade proved a turning point in the Graham Team's ministry. More than one and a half million letters were sent to Billy Graham in three months. He had been a household name for some years; now his message came right into homes across the nation. By the end of this first television crusade no less than 30,000 Americans had written in to state definite decisions made for Christ during or after the telecasts; and by the network's assessment of the normal proportion of letter-writers to viewers, the total number of decisions was probably considerably more.

From then onwards part of each crusade was televised across the nation, generally by videotape shown several weeks or months later.

Having extended beyond the original six weeks, the executive committee booked Yankee Stadium, home of the New York Yankees baseball team, for the closing rally on

July 20. The temperature inside the stadium that day was 105 degrees. More than 100,000 attended, with more thousands outside the gates, listening by loudspeaker.

Billy and the committee had already decided, after much prayer and an all-morning discussion, to extend again until August 10. Some were afraid of an anticlimax. Billy replied that he could find no Scriptural basis for troubling about that. Christ's entry into Jerusalem was a great climax; His death the following Friday was from a human viewpoint 'a great anticlimax, yet it proved to be the turning point of history.'

'Mr Graham anticipated,' wrote his secretary, Luverne Gustavson, on July 16, 'a terrible drop in attendance this week, with no large delegations booked, but it's been amazingly full! And hundreds still come forward. There is a "deeper" tone to the whole services, it seems. And Mr Graham's messages are largely to Christians, so a lot of the early converts are getting established in the Christian life. His subjects on prayer and the Holy Spirit have been exceptionally good.'

Billy was exhausted. He had been preaching ten weeks nightly without a break. He now cut out other engagements, spent most of the day in bed, sometimes would almost cling to the pulpit. 'I had nothing to give, I had exhausted my mind. Yet I'm sure that everyone would agree that the preaching had far more power. It was God taking sheer weakness – it's when I get out of the way and say, "God, You have to do it." I sat on the platform many nights with nothing to say, nothing. Just sat there. And I knew that in a few minutes I'd have to get up and preach, and I'd just say, "Oh, God, I can't do it. I cannot do it." And yet, I would stand up and all of a sudden it would begin to come – just God giving it, that's all.' The crusade cost him physically even more than London.

On August 10 they extended for the third and last time. 'Not even the most vocal critics,' Billy wrote on August 26, 'can now say that it was publicity, organization or showmanship. There is an element of the Spirit of God that is beyond analysis and rationalization.'

The crusade ended after sixteen weeks with a rally in

Times Square on the evening of Sunday, September 1.

The crowds stretched shoulder to shoulder down Broadway as far as the eye could see, and spilled into the cross streets, their singing echoing beneath the commercial buildings, hotels and movie theatres. The 'cross-roads of the world' became a great cathedral. The congregation was Graham's largest until that time, though sixteen years later in Korea he would address more than a million people face to face.

The Protestant Council of New York was in no doubt that the crusade had fulfilled its purpose. Some six months after the close its executive secretary, Dan Potter, wrote to Graham that the four objectives had been 'met in a miraculous way: to win men to Christ; to make the city God-conscious; to strengthen the churches; to make the city conscious of moral, spiritual and social responsibilities.'

On May 15, 1958, one year to the day after the opening of the crusade, the Protestant Council held a united rally at Madison Square Garden. Billy Graham sent greetings on tape from the San Francisco crusade. When the associate evangelist who was present asked converts of the previous year's crusade to stand, it seemed almost half of the 17,500 present were on their feet.

A New York minister wrote to Billy: 'The real results of the crusade are not in statistical form or in ways that can be measured. You cannot tell what the crusade did for the morale of us ministers, the new confidence it gave us, the motivation it supplies for the preaching of the Bible and Christ crucified.'

10

Under the Southern Cross

Australia did not seem to Graham the likely scene of a crusade that would move a nation. Its population was less than that of New York City and scattered over a land mass the size of the United States without Alaska. A vast preponderance lived on the Southeastern seaboard, especially around Sydney and Melbourne, but that was not immediately significant to the Team. The Australians, with an expanding economy, an exceptional emphasis on sport and the outdoor life, and a worldwide reputation for independence and bluntness of speech, had not previously proved receptive to evangelists, especially those from abroad.

The forty year old Billy came at the official invitation of the major denominations in each State, and in New Zealand, for a crusade during the late summer and autumn, February to May, 1959. Billy sent Jerry Beavan to Sydney a year earlier to prepare. Beavan soon saw that by landline relays, tape recordings, and the buying of time on radio and television, together with a full use of Operation Andrew, most of the people of Australia might be touched. 'I really believe that we are right on the verge of a national spiritual awakening here in Australia,' he wrote, 'There are so many evidences that God is doing an unusual thing that we are constantly overwhelmed by His blessing . . . There is more prayer right now in Sydney than there was in New York City at the height of that crusade.'

The first crusade was to be at Melbourne – cultured, wealthy, conservative; a quietly self-confident city that might graciously allow Graham a hearing, and little more, although the crusade chairman was Dean of the Anglican Cathedral and the vice-chairman was President-General of the Methodist Conference. For director Billy Graham sent

Walter H. Smyth, a minister from Philadelphia. Smyth had worked with him in Youth for Christ and subsequently in his film distribution office, and would take an increasingly important part in the Billy Graham ministry as International Director in the years ahead. Melbourne loved Walter for his 'brotherly and co-operative spirit', his tact and efficiency and calmness in crisis.

Early in 1959, with Australia reaching a peak of preparation, Billy was at a conference in Dallas when he began to suffer severe pain in his left eye, and restricted sight. The blockage was caused by overstrain (he might have had a thrombosis) for he had been carrying too heavy a speaking schedule, along with all the problems caused by growth of the Association. He was ordered a complete rest in the sun in Hawaii. Melbourne was postponed by a week and Sydney shortened by a week. Billy was ordered to do little more than the evening preaching, and to swim or play a short round of golf on most days.

The Australian crusade opened on February 15, 1959 at Melbourne. Despite Australian zeal, the Americans expected a small crusade, and autumn weather being chancy, had chosen the largest indoor arena (now the Festival Hall) out in West Melbourne, which seated only 7,500, increased by a temporary annex for closed circuit television to 10,000. But on the opening Sunday afternoon the arena could not contain the crowds. Billy went outside and addressed, in a sudden rainstorm, an overflow crowd estimated by the police at 5,000.

After five days the committee abandoned the arena and moved to a new open-air auditorium inaugurated the previous week, the Sidney Myer Music Bowl in King's Domain, across the Yarra River in the centre of the city. Its unusually shaped aluminium roof covered only the platform and some 2,000 seats, but the Bowl was so designed that a great audience could sit on the grass slopes and look down to the platform, and more thousands could stand behind in a wide arc. The acoustics and amplifying were perfect: the fringes of the crowd, though unable to see, could hear every word of song and sermon, and Melbourne spilled out to King's Domain in such numbers that Team and Committee marvelled at the littleness of the faith that had been content to book the indoor arena.

'When Billy gave the invitation' wrote Grady Wilson next morning, 'immediately they began streaming down the aisles from all directions. There were more than 3,000 that came forward, and finally Billy threw up his hands and said: "Stop, ladies and gentlemen, there is no more room. If you want to give your life to Christ, go home and drop me a letter in the mail and I will send you follow-up literature that will help you in your Christian life." It has been simply fantastic what God the Holy Ghost has done here.'

As hundreds of that 3,000 crowded onto the platform a hard bitten police inspector complained: 'That platform won't stand the weight, there'll be a collapse.' The inspector, who had previously indicated that the whole crusade was both nonsense and a nuisance, murmured in awed tones: 'There is something here I don't understand. There is something here with depth that is beyond me. It can only be God at work.' When numbers at the Myer Bowl on the Sunday topped 60,000 all Australia read the headlines' news of the smashing turnout.

The Music Bowl was a perfect place for the nonchurchgoer. A solicitor told a lawyer on the committee, 'I would be uncomfortable in a church, but people like me find it very easy to go along and listen to Billy in these surroundings. Everything is so natural. This is how I think Christ must have preached when He was talking to the people of His day.' Even drinkers outside a hotel called to Billy as he passed, 'Good on you, Billy, we're for you!'

Graham, Barrows and Shea had always been happy in their work, but Melbourne brought them a new happiness, all the stronger for being unexpected. Whereas New York was a battle, Melbourne and all Australia is remembered through a haze of happiness. Billy's left eye troubled him a little, but made a complete recovery. Except for the eye Billy felt fine.

The whole Team warmed to the friendliness of the Australians, as the Australians to theirs. Cliff and Bev won a large place in the affections of a nation that loves to sing. 'They created a wonderful atmosphere in the early stages of each meeting,' runs the memory of a businessman convert, 'and that atmosphere helped us to realize fully the joy and love of Christianity.'

In the third week the Myer Music Bowl had to be vacated because of Melbourne's Moomba Festival. The crusade moved to the Agricultural Showgrounds, far from the city centre and the residential suburbs – too near freight yards, power stations and a slaughter house. A third move, to uncongenial surroundings with bad acoustics, did not prove a handicap, and the crusade continued to be the main topic in Melbourne.

Then came the torrential rain of March 2. On March 3, a youth night, the rain was if possible worse, yet about 25,000 attended. The platform was not under cover. Billy's tie-microphone went out of action and he preached crouching over a low microphone on the dais. Most of the people were in the stands, but those who came forward had to plough through the mud in the open, 1,200 of them.

Meanwhile at Myer Music Bowl the rain washed away the loose earth on the slopes and poured down to flood what had been the counselling area. Had the crusade stayed it would have been drowned!

The final meeting, on Sunday, March 15, took place at the Melbourne Cricket Ground, one of the largest and best designed stadiums in the world. Long before the arrival of the governor of Victoria, Sir Dallas Brooks, the stands were full and people were still crowding into the gates. The secretary of Melbourne Cricket Club made history by allowing thousands to sit on the turf and women and children to enter the Members' Stand.

The governor read the Twenty-third Psalm and Billy, before his address, gave out a special message from President Eisenhower. Billy was overwhelmed by the size of the crowd, greater even than that of Wembley in 1954. Luverne Gustavson, far back in one of the stands, echoed the thoughts of the Team when she wrote that evening: 'It was a stirring sight to see so many people gathered so reverently for a Gospel service. Then at the end of the service when the congregation joined to sing "God be with you till we meet again", my throat got all lumpy. For

91

certainly most of these people would never meet again until in the Presence of Christ.'

More than 4,000 inquirers came forward at the invitation: with the counsellors beside them, it was an amazing sight in itself. Counselling was held up briefly when 'God Save the Queen' was played at the departure of the Queen's representative.

Even more than the governor's presence, another action seemed to spotlight Melbourne's reaction to the crusade. Close behind the Cricket Ground lies a main suburban railway. Normally, red trains and green trains clatter noisily at frequent intervals. That afternoon they were strangely muted. The committee learned afterward that the head of Victoria Railways had personally ordered trains to proceed slowly in the vicinity during the service.

Seven weeks after the Graham Team had left Melbourne, the Chief Justice of Victoria, Lieutenant-General Sir Edmund Herring, echoed in a private letter to Billy the public comments of churchmen: 'Your crusade here,' he wrote, 'has had tremendous repercussions. All the churches have new recruits to look after, and all I have been in touch with are doing everything they can to make them welcome and keep them in the fold. But, quite apart from the number of people who have either been brought into the churches or brought back to them, we all owe you a debt for sweetening our own lives and making the great bulk of the people who are, sad to say, outside the Christian World, pause and think for a minute of where they stand.' In 1964 Herring could strongly endorse his 1959 letter. 'I would say that in all sorts of ways and all sorts of places the influence of Billy Graham is still felt here.' And in 1969, in his second Melbourne Crusade, Graham could see this for himself.

After rallies in Tasmania and crusades in New Zealand – and a week's rest on Queensland beaches – Billy Graham came to Sydney for a four weeks' crusade which was firmly consolidated as part of the continuing mission of the church.

The crusade had been awaited since 1954, when the then

Archbishop of Sydney and Primate of Australia, Howard Mowll, first approached Billy Graham. Mowll, who died some months before the crusade, was so trusted that virtually the entire Protestant Church community was officially committed to support, and many individual churches and parishes shaped their programmes round it. Counselling classes enrolled more than double the number of persons that enrolled in New York, with its far greater population, though dwarfed by Los Angeles in 1963, which enrolled 23,000. Of the 6,000 people selected as counsellors or advisers, over half were Anglicans, from 160 parishes. Sydney taught the Graham Team a further new concept: the pre-crusade city-wide visitation – every home in the entire city visited with an invitation to attend.

Thousands of small prayer meetings in homes, and the press coverage from the Melbourne crusade, raised expectancy. The Sydney press had been Billy's ally ever since his first press conference on his way to Melbourne, and it covered the crusade as no other event since the Queen's visit.

On the first day 50,000 people came to the Agricultural Showground. Few of the committee had quite expected their 'city of happy pagans' to show much response, yet nearly 1,000 came forward, and so it continued day after day. From the platform it was 'always deeply moving,' writes Archbishop Marcus Loane, 'to watch the solemn audience suddenly break up when the invitation was given, like a giant human anthill stirred to life, as thousands rose from their seats in the arena or in the farthest stands to go forward.' This movement was essentially an individual action: one here, another there, pushing past the row of friends or strangers to the aisle; then, at the platform (though a host of inquirers and counsellors were all around) the convert conscious, as was often testified afterward, of no other people around. The prayer of committal would be repeated as if alone with God.

More than once heavy rain turned the Showground into a quagmire. Roy Gustafson, Billy's old friend of Florida days, had gone to Australia as his guest, 'with some big question marks. Just because numbers are large is no proof

93

that God is in it. Goliath was big . . .' On the first Friday at Sydney rain fell intermittently during the service. At the invitation, 'the rain came down like a tropical storm. You couldn't even see the people in the stands. They couldn't see the platform. And Billy started the appeal. I said to myself, "He must be crazy. No one will come tonight." But 1,700 people came, and stood in water and mud up to their ankles. I remember a counsellor drenched to the skin, with half a dozen people under an umbrella, and he in the middle standing with a Bible. Water was coming through in a fine mist and ruining the Bible, but he was pointing the half dozen to the Saviour. That night I was absolutely convinced that God had laid His hand on Billy.'

At the final service on May 10, 1959, 150,000 people were present: 80,000 in the Showground and 70,000 in the adjoining Cricket Ground, linked by amplifiers. A further one million Australians listened either by landline or by the live radio broadcast. There was an exciting touch when the two great choirs, with Bev Shea, sang 'How Great Thou Art' in alternate verses, one from the Showground, the next from the Cricket Ground. Billy preached on 'The Broad and the Narrow Way', and as the inquirers streamed forward Billy repeated, 'What a sight! what a sight, to see these hundreds coming through the rain. You who are in the Cricket Ground, you come forward too. Come and stand around the fences, and you who are listening to the landline relays, come and stand at the front of the auditorium where you are'; 5,683 people made decisions. 'The thanksgiving prayer in the follow-up room, when all the cards had come in and were being processed, was unforgettable.'

The Sydney crusade and the associate crusades which followed, with Billy travelling the continent to conclude them, stirred all Australia. As one leading minister put it succinctly and, by the evidence, accurately, 'The whole country was rocked by the Graham phenomenon.' Owing to Australia's unique distribution of population it is probable that 50 per cent heard Billy Graham in person or through landlines, and almost all the rest at least once on radio or by television. Indeed, Graham's own opinion was that it 'was through television that we most touched the major cities of Australia.'

Australia had never previously known a nationwide religious revival. The total figure of those who signified a committal to Christ in the crusade exceeded 130,000 – no less than 1.24 per cent of the population, 'a flood of new life and power into our whole religious force, which will surely go on to challenge the ungodliness and immorality about us.'

When Hugh Gough, who as Bishop of Barking had been chairman of Harringay, arrived to succeed Mowll as Archbishop of Sydney shortly after, he wrote to Billy that he was meeting hundreds of people 'who have entered into spiritual life through your crusade. Literally thousands are now being built up in the fellowship of our Anglican churches.' For the next ten years half of the members of the theological college were fruit of the crusade, directly or indirectly, whether as converts or those who came to full consecration. Missionary societies of all denominations also received scores of recruits.

Melbourne, and Sydney even more, proved how much more effective a crusade can be when, as Graham always intended, it was integrated fully into the continuing work of the churches. Whereas in New York, a year after the 1957 crusade, less than half the inquirers were found to have been contacted, the Australian churches shepherded their converts by every means available, and saw the majority become strong in faith. As the perspective of the years lengthened, 1959 stood out as a landmark date.

For Billy and the Team, 1959 ended their first ten years since Los Angeles. And gave them the assurance that in the decades ahead they 'would see greater things than these.'

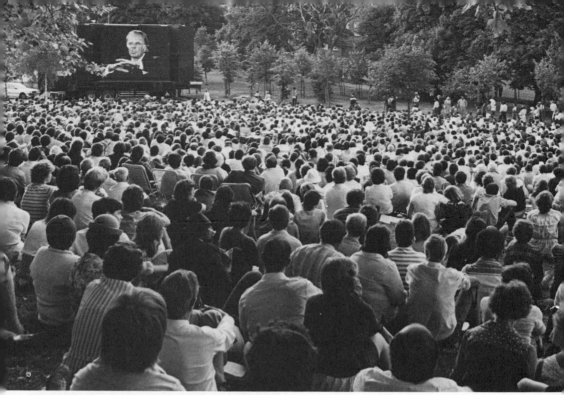

A crowd in Birmingham, England
listen to Billy by closed circuit hookup.

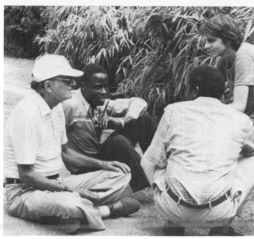

Billy during an afternoon of personal
witnessing during the
Amsterdam International Conference
of Itinerant Evangelists.

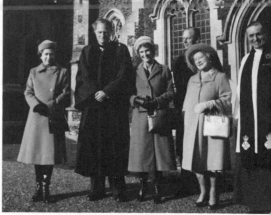

Her Majesty Queen Elizabeth II, Billy,
Ruth, His Royal Highness Prince Phillip,
the Queen Mother and the Rev. Gerry Murphy,
rector of the Sandringham parish church
in the spring of 1984.

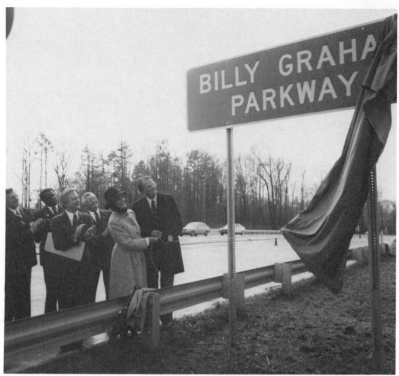

Charlotte, N.C., honors their native son, as Ruth and Billy
unveil the sign for the Billy Graham Parkway in 1983.

Billy receiving the Presidential Medal of Freedom from
President Ronald Reagan at the White House in February 1983.

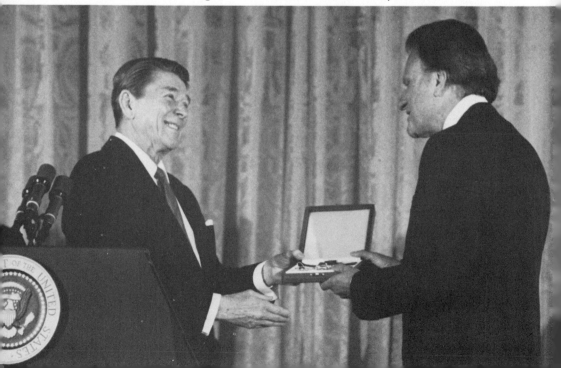

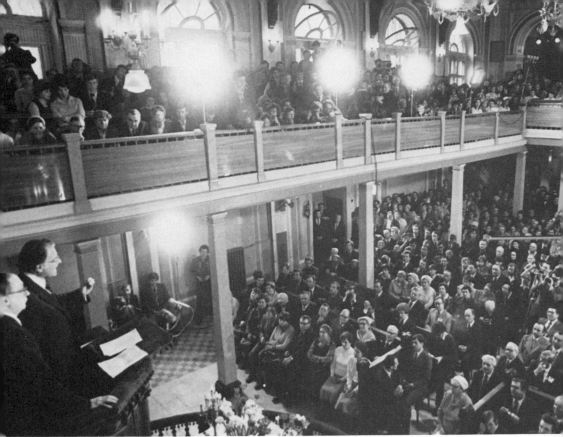

Billy preaching in the Moscow Baptist Church
during his first visit to the Soviet Union in May 1982.

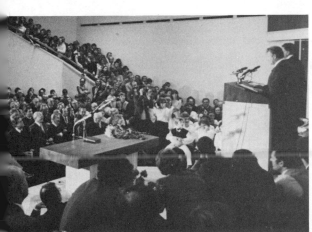

Billy before a crowd of 1200
in Bratislava, Czechoslovakia, 1982.

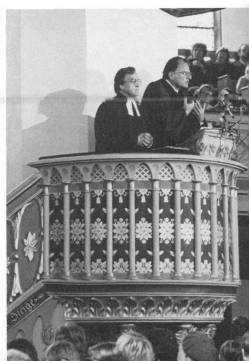

Billy in the historic Wittenburg church
pulpit, the birthplace of the Reformation,
in East Germany during a 1982 visit.

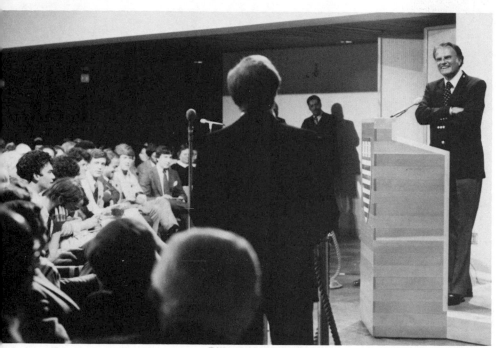

Billy enjoying lively dialogue with students at Harvard University's John F. Kennedy School of Government, 1982.

Billy informally talking to attendees of his 1982 address at Boston College.

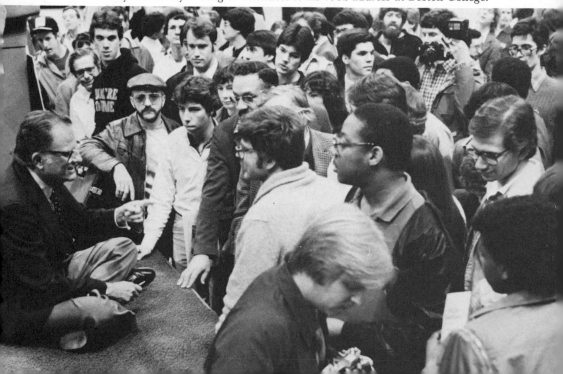

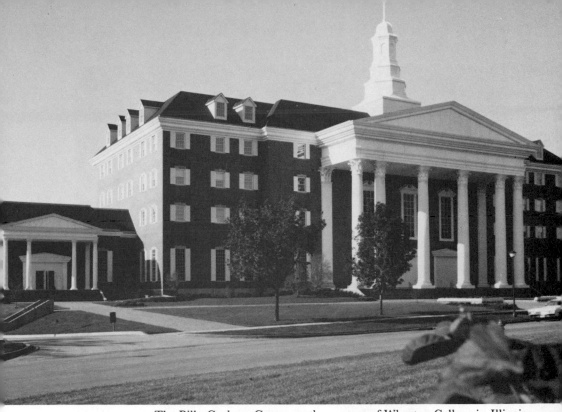

The Billy Graham Center on the campus of Wheaton College in Illinois.

Billy laying the cornerstone of the Billy Graham Center.

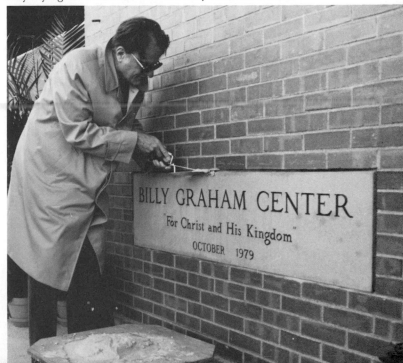

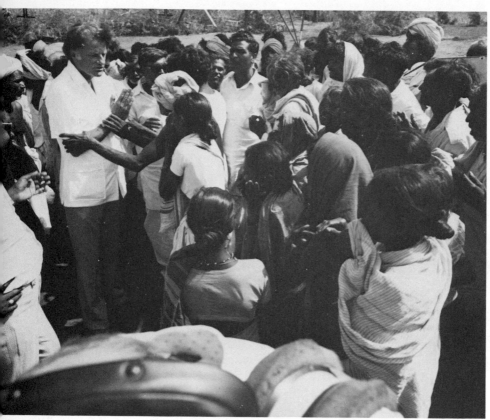

Billy encouraging the people of South India after a 1978 cyclone.

A record crowd of nearly 200,000 people gather
in Maracana Stadium in Rio de Janeiro in October 1974.

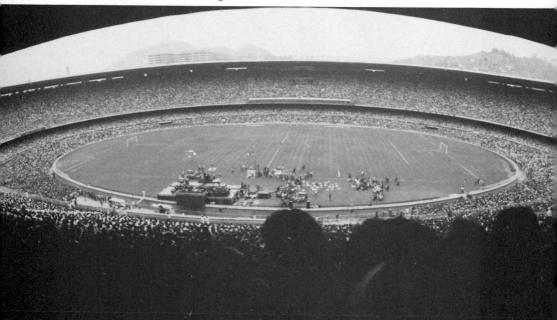

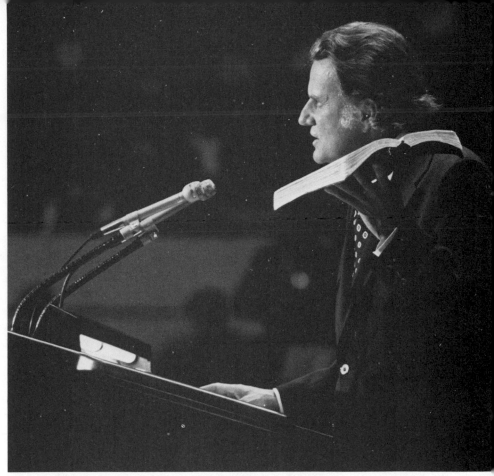

Billy, in familiar pose, as he preaches the gospel to all nations.

Conducting 1973 graveside service for President Lyndon Johnson at the Johnson Ranch in Texas.

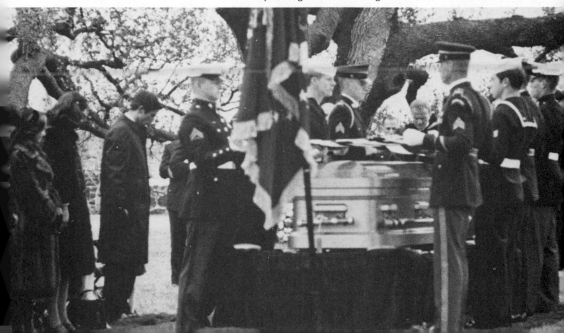

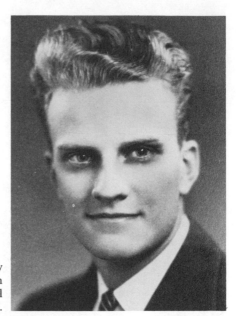

Seventeen-year-old Billy
pictured on his graduation
from the Charlotte High School
in North Carolina in June of 1935.

The tent meeting set up at Washington and Hill streets
in Los Angeles for the eight-week Greater Los Angeles Crusade in 1949.

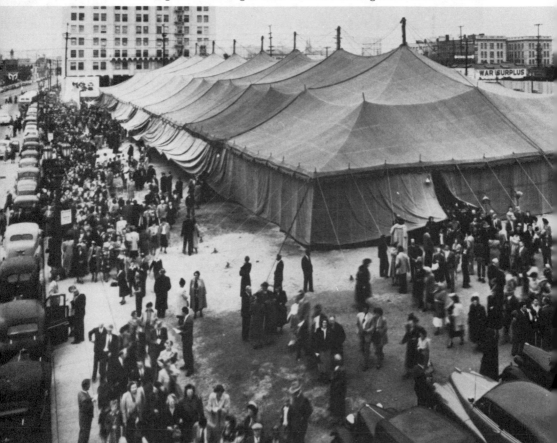

Part Two
1960–1976

11

Reaching Out

Billy and Ruth built a house in the mountains above Montreat, on land which he had bought very cheaply years earlier. Their decision that Ruth should give priority to the children, at the cost of frequent separations, brought its reward: the two sons and five daughters of the Grahams enjoyed a happy, high spirited family life despite their father's frequent absences and the pressures of his fame.

'Because of their example,' writes the eldest, Gigi, 'I respected them and listened to their advice. I saw Daddy live what he preached. I saw them making Christ their life, not just their religion.' 'I was able to see Christ in my parents,' says the youngest, Ned. 'Their love *and prayer* have guided me all my life, including my own commitment to Christ.' Franklin comments: 'History has shown that many public figures live two lives: one for the camera, the other behind closed doors. Not so with Mom and Dad. Their lives are the same before the public as they are behind closed doors.' Each of the children, in his or her time and way, dedicated their lives to Christian service and made happy marriages themselves.

From the sure base of a supremely happy home, Billy Graham's ministry expanded and deepened during the 1960s and '70s. Supported by family, Team, and the men and women of the Association offices, Billy could seize his ever widening opportunities to bring Christ's message to millions.

The years were marked by great crusades: London again, at Earl's Court; New York again, at the new Madison Square Garden; a television link-up across Europe from Dortmund, West Germany; scores of cities in North America, many capitals of the world, and some remote areas such as Nagaland.

Simultaneously, Billy was making new openings. As Ruth says, he 'is constantly thinking how best, in the short time we have left, to present the world with the claims of Christ and the hope that is to be found in the everlasting Gospel. Big thoughts. Big plans. He carries the world in his heart, as it were.'

World Wide Pictures, the motion picture arm of the Association, carried the Christian message across the continents through feature films. In America, long before the rise of the 'electronic church' Billy Graham crusades were shown regularly on television. The telecasts enormously increased the scope and results of Billy's evangelistic ministry. Some of them were later edited into films for showing in theatres and halls, while conversely the films of his crusades in distant parts were shown on television with great effect.

In 1960 he founded *Decision* magazine.

Four years earlier, with his father-in-law, Nelson Bell, he had founded *Christianity To-day* to be a 'strong, hard hitting, intellectual magazine' to propound the evangelical view. Many friends wanted Billy to make it a house organ of his Association but he decided against, and the independence of the magazine helped it to become a strong factor in the evangelical resurgence. A few years later he invited Dr Sherwood Eliot Wirt, a minister in Oakland, California who had been a journalist before ordination, and had written an excellent book about the San Francisco crusade of 1958, to create an illustrated colour magazine for popular readership. It should promote the Gospel and discipleship and bring news of the crusades and other Billy Graham ministries, so that readers would support them by prayer.

While George Wilson and the Association office in Minneapolis prepared their expansion into major magazine publishing, Woody Wirt was lent to *Christianity To-day*. 'This was good experience in editing, but totally different productionwise from what I would meet. For example, CT used no pictures. So when Billy gave me the green light at a Team meeting in Montreux in August 1960, and told me to go back to Minneapolis and put out *Decision*, I really had to start from scratch. It was on-the-job training. I had written for magazines, but knew nothing about producing one. I was a complete and total ignoramus! The one thing I did know was good writing from poor, and I determined that *Decision* should have no mediocre material.

'I visited New York and talked to religion editors of various media. I remember old Dr Bradbury, the editor of the Baptist *Watchman–Examiner*, whom I visited in his funny little office high in an old building in Manhattan. I asked him what he thought *Decision* should be like and he said, "Mr Wirt, there is a hiatus in the field of Christian publishing. We used to emphasize Christ and His work and the Holy Spirit, and what it means to walk with God. Our magazines don't do that any more and it's a pity." I thought, "By the grace of God, that's the kind of magazine I want to put out."

'So instead of talking about the ramifications of the Christian faith, *Decision* talked about the faith itself, its source, its meaning, its significance. We talked about grace, and faith, and the cross, and the Bible, and especially about Jesus. We tried in every issue to show how people could be saved. And I soon struck a principle of balance.'

Each issue would include a sermon by Billy Graham, stories from his latest crusade and a focus on prayer for the next. In another popular feature men and women told how they had found Christ through the Graham ministries and of how their lives had changed: *Decision* selected a few representative stories each month from the flood of letters which poured unsolicited into Minneapolis. They were selected to help others, not to glorify Graham.

The balance would be made up with a Bible Study; articles for youth; for women; articles about history or biography and to feature the missionary call. 'I also went for the light touch and for poetry. Russ Busby's photos and Bob Blewett's paintings made a great contribution. In time we assimilated a fine staff and the production of the magazine became a thrilling experience. We had wonderful support from Billy, from the Team, and from the staff and employees at the Minneapolis office. As for the readers, it was simply amazing to see the subscriptions come in every day by the hundreds. We seldom got a critical letter.'

Decision carried no advertisements yet paid its way from the start. Within nine years the circulation in North America had reached four million. Before its twentieth birthday *Decision* in its different editions and in six languages had become monthly reading in five continents. Sherwood Wirt and, after his retirement, Roger Palms have kept it a force for Christ across the world.

Billy was quick to accept and absorb the suggestions of others. The late Lowell Berry, an industrialist of San Francisco whose life had been blessed by the crusade of 1958, suggested that a school of evangelism should be held during a crusade. In the fourteen years after the first school, held during the Chicago crusade of 1962, Berry gave half a million dollars in scholarships.

The schools have become one of the most significant segments of the Billy Graham ministry.[1] They have been of incalculable influence on pastors and students. For an example: the school held during the Rio de Janeiro crusade of 1974. It drew some 3,500 men and women to Rio. They came from Amazon rain forests and the cool southern mountains, from the savannahs, from new Brasilia and teeming Sao Paulo, travelling by country bus along earth roads and then by swift modern buses along the network of highways that link the enormous country. From Recife, with its glorious beaches, a convoy of four buses included most of the Baptist seminary and the women's college for Christian education, both drawing their students from throughout the northeast. They travelled night and day for forty-two hours, to hear 'a great and famous preacher', to 'learn his methods', to 'share in the work of the crusade'.

The Brazilians appreciated every lecture, but the seminars were the high spots. These gave time to talk and discover one another, for most of them knew little or nothing of Christians in other denominations. The school of evangelism broke down those barriers throughout Brazil, just as the crusade preparations had broken barriers in

1. For more detail about their origin see *Evangelist to the World* pp 130–132.

Greater Rio. The atmosphere of the school, its spirituality and the seriousness with which it faced the problems of evangelism, heartened pastors and laity, especially the young.

Billy Graham and the crusade itself formed the focal points. When Billy addressed the school, his evangelistic emphasis and his appeal for a deep spiritual life left a strong impression. A pastor in the rolling uplands of Minas Gerais, living four hours' bus ride from the regional city and forty minutes walk from the bus stop, summed up the school of evangelism: 'It all really boils down to one thing: I got out of the school of evangelism a passion for souls.'

The pastors from the interior, like those of Rio who had prepared the crusade, were heartened and humbled when they attended the huge stadium services, especially the final Sunday afternoon with its extraordinary atmosphere of joy. They watched in awe the 225,000 who had gathered to hear Billy, for the total of non-Catholics in Rio in 1974 numbered less than 100,000. They heard the hammering on the gates, as the service began, by those who could not get in.

And when they returned home they were at once able to put into practice what they had learned, for the whole service had been televised live: the television company estimated that 25 million people had watched and heard Billy's sermon.

12

The Reconciler

In September 1963 a Baptist church in a black area of Birmingham, Alabama, was destroyed by bombs which caused the death of four children. It was one more serious incident in the racial tension of those years in the southern states of America.

The next Easter Day, 1964, Billy Graham brought his Team, which had been racially integrated for seven years, for an evangelistic rally in Birmingham's main stadium, where the segregation between blacks and whites, then customary, was abandoned for the day. Bev Shea recalls the fear of many in the city that such a move would provoke violence, but the community leaders believed that Billy Graham could have a deeper impact than any one else.

The crowd of over 30,000, estimated to be about equally black and white, went out of its way to be friendly to one another. Graham preached a straight address of love, repentance and faith, and the national press reporters were stunned at the response, as blacks and whites streamed forward at the invitation.

Billy Graham was able to promote racial conciliation because he had been among the first to do so, and had worked consistently for the end of segregation in the South. As a southern boy he had taken it for granted. 'It rarely occurred to me in my childhood to think about the difficulties, problems, and oppressions of black people. In high school, I began to question some of the practices, but it was not until I'd actually committed my life to Christ that I began to think more deeply about it.' At Wheaton, which had been founded as an anti-Slavery school and was 'very strong in its social conscience, especially on the race question, I began to realize for the first time that if I were a Christian, I had to take a stand.'

More than forty years later, at the Tacoma crusade of 1983, a black woman who came from the South told the local newspaper about her childhood memory of the young unknown Billy Graham. He was to be the preacher at a tent revival during his vacation from Wheaton. She was with her mother and the other coloured people (as they were then known) at the back, segregated behind the customary rope. While they waited, the child of her mother's white employers came down to play with her and they strayed from the rope as they played. A white woman checked her. 'She was propelling me towards the back of the tent,' recalls the Tacoma resident, when a large hand settled on her shoulder. It was Billy Graham.

'You're going the wrong way, sister,' he said. 'She belongs down front – all the children belong down front so God can smile on them.'

'He gently loosened me from the woman's grip and led both of us children to the front of the tent. Then he had all the children, coloured and white, gathered at the front of the tent. The segregation rope was removed, because Billy Graham refused to preach to a segregated audience.'

When he first began crusades in the South, in 1950, Billy accepted segregation in seating but not among those who came forward: 'There's no racial distinction here,' he would say from the podium. 'The ground is level at the foot of the cross.' At a southern crusade in 1952 he personally pulled down the ropes. 'That was among my first acts of conscience on the race question. I determined from then on I would never preach to another segregated audience.'

The Chattanooga crusade of 1953, more than a year before the Supreme Court Judgement of 1954, was fully integrated, and every crusade afterwards.

In 1956, after a private talk with President Eisenhower, Graham went quietly to work among religious leaders of both races in the South, encouraging them individually to take a stronger stand for desegregation and yet to demonstrate charity and patience. During the following years he went at personal risk to flash points in the racial conflict to hold integrated meetings of reconciliation in the aftermath of violence. President Johnson wrote to him:

105

'You are doing a brave and fine thing for your country in your courageous effort to contribute to the understanding and brotherhood of the Americans in the South.'

By pen and speech Graham supported civil rights reform, but he would not join freedom marches, convinced that he could contribute a better way. He was abused by both sides in the conflict.

Martin Luther King understood and appreciated Billy Graham's work. In 1957 Graham invited King to brief the Team. During the New York crusade King addressed them twice privately and sat on the platform one evening. In later years the two men twice held long discussions and in 1960, at the world Baptist conference in Rio de Janeiro, Billy gave a dinner in Martin Luther King's honour, inviting Southern Baptist leaders, some of whom were uncomfortable at eating with King, since restaurants, toilets, hotels, and most churches, were segregated in the South at that time. In his speech at the dinner King said that his work for civil rights would be much harder were it not for the Graham crusades.

Graham was certain that the race problem was fundamentally moral and spiritual. Forced changes on either side would deepen prejudice, 'But if you preach the love of Christ and the transforming power of Christ, there is not only a spiritual change but a psychological and moral change. The man who receives Christ forgets all about race when he is giving his life to Christ.'

An outstanding example was Jimmy Karam of Little Rock, Arkansas, who had become notorious in the nation as a violent leader of those who resisted federal attempts to impose integration in the schools. A lapsed Catholic, married to a Baptist; successful businessman; political boss: 'I was a real rough, tough fellow.' On a visit to New York in 1957 Karam was taken against his will by Governor Forbush to the Billy Graham crusade. He heard Billy say that it made no difference what sort of life you had lived. Christ had died for your sins, and risen from the dead; therefore God can wipe the slate clean if you will believe.

'If Billy Graham had said that night, "Now, Jimmy, you have got to quit drinking: you have got to quit gambling and running around, and lying," I would have said, "Forget it. I have been trying to quit. There is no way." I had tried all of my life to live a decent life. But when I accepted Jesus Christ into my life, he took away drinking, smoking, gambling, running around and all the things I couldn't do for myself. He did it just like that. That is what is so wonderful about Christ. That is what is so wonderful about Billy Graham's ministry. I don't care how many kings or queens he had been with, Billy Graham has saved lives such as mine all over the world. And that is what he lives for; he lives to see lost people find salvation through Christ and then to help us grow in Christ.'

Jimmy Karam's family soon saw that he had stopped swearing but his reputation was so terrible that his daughter's pastor declined to waste time counselling him; then the pastor came, saw his sincerity and helped him to consolidate the decision. Karam quickly became a force for racial conciliation in the South and for evangelism. 'My whole life changed. I only wanted to tell other people about Christ. Every talk I make is my testimony of what my life was before Christ and what it now is with Christ.' Being of Lebanese origin he can speak with authority about the tensions between Arabs and Jews, between whites and blacks, which only Christ can give strength to resolve.

Karam and his pastor, W. O. Vaught, wanted to bring Graham to Little Rock. Local conditions made this impossible for two years. Then a week that began with yet another bombing ended with meetings in War Memorial Stadium, which led Vaught, the crusade chairman, to write to Billy: 'There has been universal agreement in all the churches and out across the city that your visit here was one of the finest things that ever happened in the history of Little Rock. So very many people have changed their attitude, so many people have washed their hearts of hatred and bitterness, and many made decisions who had never expected to make such decisions.'

Many years later, when Martin Luther King was dead but violence and discrimination had disappeared from the southern states, Senator Daniel Moynihan summed up well in a private letter to Billy: 'You and Rev King, more than any two men – and, surely, with God's help – brought your own South out of that long night of racial fear and hate.'

But Billy was not concerned for his own country only. He worked for racial reconciliation in the Middle East and wherever he had opportunity. Nowhere was this more evident than in South Africa. He refused to conduct a crusade or rally unless apartheid conditions were lifted.

The opportunity came at last in 1973 through the work of Michael Cassidy, a South African brought to Christ at Cambridge University through a friend who had been converted at Harringay. Billy's 1955 mission at Cambridge followed soon afterwards and Michael had a new hero. At the New York crusade in 1957 he dedicated his life to mass evangelism in Africa. He founded Africa Enterprise.

By 1973 Cassidy was able to promote an inter-racial, integrated Congress of evangelism at Durban, which Billy Graham addressed. At King's Park rugby stadium in Durban on Sunday afternoon of the Congress, and at Wanderer's cricket ground in Johannesburg a week later, Billy preached to completely integrated audiences.

At Durban, so quiet and good-natured was the crowd that the police dogs which were usually needed to separate brawlers when different races came in big numbers to a stadium, were soon returned to the vans. The police kept out of sight. Apartheid had even been lifted from the toilets. The friendliness of the races, their discovery of each other as being equally first-class citizens made a startling impact on Durban, especially because of the immense size of the rally; even opponents recognized that only Billy Graham could have brought it together in the South Africa of 1973.

'The sight of black and white South Africa together in that field,' said a black bishop, 'singing and praying to the one God, was a foretaste of what future generations in this land are certain to enjoy if we today will be faithful.'

At Johannesburg, where the sermon was carried live to the whole nation by South African radio, the conclusion of Billy's sermon brought an immediate response. In the cricket ground, what at first seemed a sprinkle of individuals became a slow floodtide of humanity. The platform where Billy stood waiting, chin on hand in prayer,

108

had been set in the centre of a counselling circle, fifty yards wide, reached by aisles kept open between the massed listeners sitting on the turf in front of the packed-out stands. The inquirers, pressing forward, filled the counselling space, yet still came down the aisles in a great flow of all colours of face and clothing.

Less than 3,000 trained counsellors helped more than 4,000 people who had streamed to the front. Separated peoples, from every race in South Africa, mingled. The fear that lies at the root of apartheid was lost at the foot of the Cross.[1]

1. A full account of Billy Graham's South African visit is in *Evangelist to the World*, Chapter 3.

13

Scenes from East and West

In August 1963 Billy Graham held a crusade in Los Angeles, where he had sprung to fame fourteen years before. Instead of the circus style tent of 1949 the Team had the Los Angeles Coliseum, America's largest stadium, used primarily for football and track meets, a vast oval with the tiers rising sheer from ground level.

On one youth night the number who came forward (3,216) did not fall much short of the aggregate of decisions recorded in the entire eight weeks of Los Angeles '49. Despite the huge crowds, the reverent dignity was unforgettable. 'I can't get over it,' exclaimed the comedian Jack Benny. 'These people are so quiet! I have never seen anything like it.'

At the final service 134,254 persons passed through the turnstiles, leaving an estimated 20,000 outside; the highest number recorded for any event at the Coliseum. The Stadium later erected a bronze plaque recording the occasion, bearing in bas-relief Graham's head and an impression of the scene.

After Cliff had led the choir and people in song, and Bev Shea had brought all to a quiet expectancy by his solo before the sermon, Billy Graham once again set forth the essentials of the Christian Gospel. Then he said: 'I'm going to ask you to do something tough and hard, I'm going to ask you to get up out of your seat, hundreds of you, get up out of your seat, and come out on this field and stand here reverently. Say tonight, "I do want Christ to forgive me, I want a new life, I want to live clean and wholesome for Christ, I want Him to be my Lord and my Master." God has spoken to you. You get up and come – we're going to wait right now – quickly – hundreds of you from everywhere.'

And not another word. He stood back, arms folded, head bent in prayer. At once the flow began. As in Sydney or Chicago or scores of cities throughout the world, it looked from the platform like a mass movement; but far up in the stadium it was one here, another there – a deliberate, costly choice, down the aisles and across the ramps over the race track and onto the grass. Billy Graham stands motionless, a distant figure barely discernible above the sea of people, young and old; waiting until the tide ceases to flow and he can address them briefly before the benediction is given and the counselling begins.

On the platform one night sat the German theologian, Professor Helmut Thielicke of Hamburg, who had come frankly critical. But he 'saw it all happen without pressure and emotionalism (contrary to the reports which I had received up until now) . . . I saw them all coming towards us, I saw their assembled, moved and honestly decided faces, I saw their searching and their meditativeness. I confess that this moved me to the very limits. Above all there were two young men – a white and a black – who stood at the front and about whom one felt that they were standing at that moment on Mount Horeb and looking from afar into a land they had longed for. I shall never forget those faces. It became lightning clear that men *want* to make a decision . . .'

'The consideration that many do not remain true to their hour of decision can contain no truly serious objection; the salt of this hour will be something they will taste in every loaf of bread and cake which they are to bake in their later life. *Once* in their life they have perceived what it is like to enter the realm of discipleship. And if only this memory accompanies them, then that is already a great deal. But it would certainly be more than a mere memory. It will remain an appeal to them, and in this sense it will maintain its character *indelibilis*.'

Billy and the Team were determined to do all that they could to lessen the number of those who did not 'remain true to their hour of decision'. Training and follow up were useless without prayer, but with prayer and profound trust in the Holy Spirit the Team continually refined, improved and adapted the methods which they offered to the churches. Thus, as the decades passed, a crusade could handle numbers which would have been unbelievable in the earlier years.

The crusade at Seoul in the Republic of Korea in 1973 dwarfed the numbers recorded at Los Angeles ten years earlier.

In the wide Han River which marks the western edges of down-town Seoul lies the open space of Yoido island where Samuel Moffett, the first missionary, had landed in 1883 and was stoned; one of the stone-throwers became a convert and the first to go as a missionary to his own people. Yoido is linked to each bank by bridges carrying the main road to the airport. The island's chief feature is the 'May 16' People's Plaza, a long narrow paved runway, approximately one mile by 200 yards, formerly the famous 'Quay 16' landing ground of the Korean War. This was the place secured for the crusade.

About 300,000 people gathered for the first service: the ground had been grid-marked for crowd control, allowing almost exact statistics. As Team and staff members looked from the platform at the crowd stretching away in both directions of the long Plaza, some wept openly as they felt 'the waves of anticipation and joy and excitement pouring up' from that huge crowd down below. Long-serving missionaries like Sam Moffett, son of that first missionary, had been expecting a multitude yet he was 'stunned by the emotional impact of that many people on that island.' Graham had often said that statistics are totally meaningless in the sight of God but no preacher could fail to be moved when he walked onto the platform and saw such a crowd under the arc lights. Ruth wrote to her family, 'It is one of those things impossible to take in.'

Throughout the crusade great numbers of Koreans spent all night in prayer on the Plaza, while others prayed in the churches. Pastors stoked the fires: 'I continued,' recalls one, 'to emphasize three things in my church. First, prayer. Second, attendance by all members at the crusade. Third, I encouraged them to take their unsaved friends.' The crusade became the talk of the city from cabinet minister to waitress, shop assistant and barber. It was a chief topic on talk shows and the news. Friday was Army Night and Saturday Youth Night. Christians, excited at the huge numbers attending, began to aim at no less than a million for the closing service on Sunday afternoon. That would be a resounding witness to both parts of the divided nation. At the committee's request Billy Graham publicly suggested that for the glory of God it would be wonderful to have a million to hear the Gospel face to face.

Billy was determined that it should be for God's glory, not the Team's. As one missionary commented: 'Here were men and women who were really committed to the things of God. It became very obvious to me why He was blessing their ministry so richly: it was because they had no illusions but that it was all his. They seemed very careful from Mr Graham on down, to protect that aspect and not to get their eyes off Jesus – less, like Peter, they sink into the waves.'

Sunday 3 June 1973 turned warm with only passing clouds. Two hours before the service timed for three pm, Graham and his interpreter, Dr Billy Kim, joined the stream flowing toward Yoido.

When Graham mounted the platform a solid block of humanity quietly awaited him. Every section, every aisle between, and away to edges of the Plaza hitherto unused, sat an unbroken mass of people, who throughout that service, unless singing, stayed incredibly quiet. In Kim's experience of Korean crowds none had been so still. Even children seemed neither to fidget nor cry. Statistically there should have occurred hundreds of faintings, dozens of heart attacks or other medical emergencies, yet the first-aid posts dealt with a mere 117 minor cases. Dissidents or protesters or cranks might have abounded, yet only one mental case made a brief commotion close to the platform.

The grid chart registered the figure of one million, one hundred and twenty thousand present. Korean Christians and Team alike felt that organization, publicity, a famous preacher could not have drawn that crowd and kept it so reverent. 'It had to be the Holy Spirit.' Many had waited all night and then through a hot morning. One bedridden old lady, nearing death and forbidden by her family to go, crawled out of her bedroom window and dragged herself to the Plaza.

For all who took part, that final crusade service is a dream-like memory: the solemn responsibility of ministering to such a multitude, the visual impact of so many mortals in one place.

Billy Graham knew he had a special responsibility when he came to the invitation at the close of his sermon. With a million present it would have been easy to trigger a mass reaction. He therefore made his invitation harder than usual. 'If you're willing to *forsake all other gods*, stand up.' There was a hush upon the audience at first. Then one here and one there arose, until thousands were standing. Billy led them in the prayer of accepting Christ. He gave them his brief word on the duties and responsibilities of a Christian. Then he said, 'Counsellors with your material, make your way back to those people who are standing.' Over 12,000 cards came in that day. Thousands more followed by mail from persons contacted without time for proper counselling. And, as the future showed, a great many made genuine commitments who never were reached by a counsellor at the Plaza.

The million did not move during the counselling. Many prayed as they sat. Thousands upon thousands began to sing. Then a helicopter rose from behind the platform. Dr Han, the chairman, put up his hand for silence. He explained that Billy Graham was leaving Korea that afternoon and he could not say goodbye personally to everybody but his helicopter would circle in farewell over the Plaza.

At Dr Han's word, the entire million and more stood and waved their hymnsheets or newspapers or whatever they carried. It was unbelievably poignant. Billy found the breathtaking view of this waving multitude indescribable: 'The only comment I have is, "Thanksgiving to God for all He did!"'[1]

1. A fuller account of the Korean crusade is in *Evangelist to the World*, Chapters 4 and 5.

14

True Friendship

America was in uproar over Watergate in the spring of 1973.

When Billy Graham returned to North Carolina for the Charlotte crusade between his work in South Africa and that in Korea, he was pressed to comment on television and in print. His views were widely quoted.

'Of course, I have been mystified and confused and sick about the whole thing as I think every American is,' he said. He called for punishment of the guilty and replacement of 'everybody connected with Watergate', but deplored trial by the media and by rumour, and leaks of confidential evidence. He saw the scandal as 'a symptom of the deeper moral crisis ... The time is overdue for Americans to engage in some deep soul-searching about the underpinnings of our society and our goals as a nation.' No political party could claim to be 'Mr Clean'.

Graham did not then think that President Nixon had known about Watergate, believing that 'his moral and ethical principles wouldn't allow him to do anything illegal like that. I've known him a long time and he has a very strong sense of integrity.'

Richard Nixon and Billy Graham had in fact been friends for over twenty years. 'The friendship is well rooted,' wrote Nixon's daughter, Julie Nixon Eisenhower, in 1975, 'and stems from the days when my grandmother first began to follow the ministry of Dr Graham. I am sure that part of my father's feeling that he can trust Billy Graham as a man of God stems from his knowledge that Nana believed with all her heart in the Graham mission.'

The friendship grew deeper during the years when Nixon was vice-president, for President Eisenhower had great affection for Graham, and in the Kennedy-Johnson

115

period.[1] In December 1967 Nixon begged Billy, who was convalescent after pneumonia, to join him in Florida where he had gone alone to decide whether to seek the Republican nomination for 1968. As they walked the sands together Graham glimpsed Nixon's fear of the pain and trouble the Presidency would bring; but the 1970s would be dangerous for America and the world, and Nixon believed he could contribute. Graham's counsel was a strong factor in Nixon's decision to run.

Graham was not partisan. Lyndon Baines Johnson trusted him and was the first to attend a Graham crusade while President. After laying down office, LBJ recalled 'those lonely occasions at the White House when your prayers and your friendship helped to sustain a President in an hour of trial . . . No one will ever know how you helped to lighten my load or how much warmth you brought into our house. But I know.' Mrs Lady Bird Johnson shared with the present writer her feelings of affection for Billy and Ruth Graham. 'I know how much Lyndon treasured Dr Graham's counsel. He found solace in him both as a religious adviser and a friend in good times and in times of trial and anguish. My appreciation for them has grown through the years – for the ways in which they have touched and enriched our lives and the lives of people the world over.'

In the election of 1968, when Nixon realized that he had won by a hairsbreadth, he invited Graham to his hotel suite, called his family together and asked Graham to lead them in a prayer before he went down to meet the press. Billy thought this rather significant because the President-elect, of Quaker background, had been reluctant to talk openly about his personal faith – though Graham believed it to be deep.

When forming the new administration Nixon asked Billy Graham what job he would like. Graham replied, 'You could not offer me a job as an ambassador, or a cabinet post, that I would give a second thought to. When God called me

1. For Graham's relations with Presidents Eisenhower, Kennedy and Johnson, see *Evangelist to the World*, Chapter 14.

to preach, it was for life.' Nixon said, 'I knew you would say that, and I respect you for it.' The press built up Billy as if he and his ideals were a major influence behind the Nixon White House. His influence in fact counted for less than was popularly supposed. He was one of a wide range of clergy asked to preach. He saw the President on fewer occasions privately than he had President Johnson, and knew less of what went on. The Grahams were given to understand that some of the White House staff were anxious to restrict and frustrate any influence he might have.

Nevertheless the two men remained friends in spite of the inevitably changed relationship when a private citizen becomes President. Like millions of Americans, Billy Graham's feelings toward the Nixon of 1969–71 were positive.

Nixon attended the Knoxville crusade in 1970, and his presence provoked anti-war protests. When Charlotte honoured Billy Graham in 1971 President Nixon, then at a peak of achievement nationally and internationally, 'gave one of the finest non-political addresses I've ever heard,' wrote the day's organizer, who added: 'The President spoke without notes and quite obviously from the heart in a moving tribute to Billy.' In January 1973, during celebrations following the second inaugural after Nixon's landslide victory, Billy noticed a slight change in the President. 'I could tell by his eyes that he was under some severe strain. At that time I had no idea what was about to come, nor did any of his other friends.'

The emerging Watergate scandal dismayed and shocked Graham.

During the summer of his return from Korea he found the political situation 'so discouraging that it has almost made me physically sick.' He wrote: 'While I cannot defend the Nixon administration's wrongdoing, I am disturbed by the "overkill".' He believed that America harmed itself by a double standard which condoned lawbreaking by men with more popular causes.

Graham was attacked by those who held that 'though supposedly a "moral leader", he failed to cut bait with the immorality of the White House until it was too late and any criticism of Nixon would seem to be like kicking a friend when he was down.' Many who admired Graham were puzzled by his refusal to condemn; at the same time he was being urged by those who stood by Nixon to rally publicly to his defence. 'He was criticized severely' one of Graham's oldest friends recalls, 'but once again it was his love for a friend he was seeking to help, in his onerous task as President – a friend, rightly or wrongly, who was going through a tough time.'

Graham, however, was unable to get through to the President. During the 1972 campaign a White House staffer had suggested a debate between an opposition candidate and Graham; the President killed the idea: 'No, it may hurt his ministry.' 'That was his general attitude throughout my years of friendship,' comments Graham, who believed that for such a reason Nixon deliberately kept aloof as the crisis deepened. 'I tried to get in touch with him a number of times, to assure him of my prayers and urge him to seek the Lord's guidance in a very difficult situation . . . Mr Nixon was a personal friend and at no time did I consider him as a parishioner. I seriously doubt if he looked upon me as his pastor, though having a pastor's heart (even though I am an evangelist) my feelings could not help but go out to him in his times of suffering and sorrow. There was little I could do for him except pray.'

In December he was invited to preach at the White House and they had a long private talk. While in Washington Graham recorded a candid and perceptive discussion of his views which *Christianity To-day* published in January 1974. The two men met once and talked on the telephone twice in the six weeks following publication. 'I am sure,' wrote Graham, 'that he understands that we cannot condone the things that are wrong, even though we love him as a friend and respect him as a world leader. At the same time I am well aware of the forces that are arrayed against him. I am convinced that he will survive.'

Then, in May 1974, came the Watergate tapes. They revealed a man who was a stranger to Graham. It seemed almost as if there were two personalities in one skin: the man he had known and the totally different man of the tapes; Graham repudiates the view that Nixon fraudulently hid his character to maintain their friendship.

'The whole situation,' says Ruth Graham, 'was the hardest thing that Bill has ever gone through personally.' With great reluctance Graham issued a statement condemning the blasphemies and repudiating the behaviour, but refusing to forsake Nixon, for which he was heavily criticized.

When the climax came, Graham was in Europe for his long prepared Lausanne Congress, and then in hospital with an infected jaw-bone. Thus he was spared the deepest agonies of the President's personal friends. After the resignation, Graham's efforts to speak personally or on the telephone were rebuffed until a telephone conversation in November.

In March 1975, shortly before the Albuquerque crusade, Billy Graham was invited to San Clemente. 'The purpose of the visit,' writes Julie Eisenhower, 'was simply to reassure both of my parents of his complete love and faith in them. The lack of hypocrisy and absence of a "holier than thou" attitude had always impressed me tremendously. Dr Graham's capacity for friendship and his eagerness to love make him stand apart from other men.'

Watergate was a deep shadow and disappointment to Graham but it highlighted his compassion and integrity. 'A real friend,' commented George Cornell of Associated Press, 'remains one in a pinch, particularly so then; and any friendship is hollow and a sham if it doesn't stand up under pressure, when trouble comes. Personally, my hat is off to Graham for continuing to be a friend when being so was rough and when expediency was against it. A weaker character would turn tail when a friend starts going under, afraid of getting bruised himself in the downfall.'

The crusades which followed showed Billy Graham's strength to be undiminished. And Watergate must be seen in perspective. It finished and was past just as Billy Graham reached a new plateau. Through the Lausanne Congress on World Evangelization and all that followed, he was beginning a world ministry on a wider scale than ever before.

15

Lausanne

On 16 July 1974 nearly 4,000 people from more than 150 nations gathered in the Palais de Beaulieu at Lausanne, Switzerland. The opening fanfare rang through the convention hall, hung with banners which displayed in six languages the motto of the Congress, *Let the Earth Hear His Voice*.

The climax of the first evening was a major address from Billy Graham. Billy knew the urgency of the hour. He believed in the possibility of world evangelization by the end of the twentieth century. He could help Christ's church on earth recover, in the century's last quarter, the thrust and passion that had been lost in its first. His speech 'raised high the banner of true evangelical, Biblical Christianity. It made very clear the issues of our day, and what Lausanne was and where it was going. Everyone was thrilled with this bold, forthright declaration of contemporary evangelical truth.'

Immediately after his address Billy Graham and Bishop Jack Dain, the Congress executive chairman, switched on the 'Population Clock'. Placed in a huge illuminated map of the world, this clicked up the net number being born. A few moments later the figure had reached 25; by 9.55 pm that evening it showed 163,569. When formally switched off it had registered that over 1,800,000 persons in need of the Christian Gospel had been born since the Congress began.

The Lausanne Congress had grown from a seed bed planted by Billy sixteen years earlier when he had brought a small group to another Swiss resort to discuss the urgency and issues of world evangelization. From that had come a World Congress in Berlin in 1966. The Emperor Haile Selassie of Ethiopia opened it with a resounding call: 'O Christians, let us arise and, with spiritual zeal and earnestness which characterized the apostles and the early Christians, let us labour to lead our brothers and sisters to our Saviour Jesus Christ who only can give life in its fullest sense.' A few years later, overthrown by a Marxist coup, he was put in prison and died.

The twelve hundred delegates reflected the pattern of the times, the majority being born in the West although many served developing nations. The Congress demonstrated that those who accepted the authority of Scripture and believed in leading others to the living Christ were far greater in numbers, learning and influence than had been supposed. To the Church as a whole, absorbed in concern for restructuring society, building unity or redefining belief, Berlin brought an urgent, considered appeal 'to return to a dynamic zeal for world evangelism.'

Berlin gave rise to regional congresses which had immense effect throughout the world. They were financed by the BGEA but Billy kept away, 'for fear that they would think I was in a dominant role.'

By January 1970 he had seen the need for a second world congress, to discuss and carry forward all the implications of Christ's Great Commission to His disciples. Billy moved slowly. Once the decision was made the preparation was thorough, and thus the Lausanne Congress of July 1974 made an immediate decisive impact on those who attended.

From the outset they sensed that it ushered in a new epoch. The division between missionary-sending and missionary-receiving nations had gone. Whites were outnumbered; skin colour was insignificant in this totally interracial Congress 'magnificently obsessed' with reaching the unreached in a spirit of love.

The Third World was not looking in on the deliberations of the West, as at Berlin, but giving counsel and inspiration equally: a person's contribution, not background, counted. Those who lived in spiritual backwaters like Britain and Western Europe were surprised to find how fast Christianity grew elsewhere. A Bolivian bishop wrote afterward to Billy that he and his countrymen had 'not only received inspiration and challenge and a large amount of materials for our task today, but also the evidence of the amazing renewal of the churches of Christ around the world.'

The participants found that this Congress was moulded by their own hard work and deliberations. Unlike many international church conferences, no secretariat sought to impose theologies or conclusions, nor did they need to wrest its direction from the hands of any dominant faction. Lausanne achieved a fusion of minds, hearts and aims, because it was not afraid of tensions.

In no area was participation more evident than in the creation of the Lausanne Covenant, a term chosen deliberately. 'We wanted to do more than find an agreed formula of words: we were determined not just to declare something but to do something, namely to commit ourselves to the task of world evangelization.' The long, closely argued Lausanne Covenant was an authentic act of those gathered there. Therefore it was taken seriously and studied carefully at Geneva, Lambeth, Rome and throughout the Christian world. Evangelicals were soon acting on it, as Billy Graham could comment four months later: 'It seems that God inspired a historic document that could well be a theological watershed for evangelicals for generations to come.'

The Congress also set up the Lausanne Continuation Committee. In the years which followed, this sponsored work shops and conferences on matters of great moment, and research; it forged new methods and understandings for the fulfilling of the Lausanne Covenant and the Great Commission from which the Covenant derived.

For most of the eight days at the Palais de Beaulieu Billy Graham stayed in the background. Dain writes, 'He was always available for consultation, guidance and advice without ever seeking to intrude his role into that of the Congress itself. He was the honorary chairman and yet he was very, very rarely seen on the platform. In itself this is a remarkable tribute to a man of God who has wielded, under God, such power and influence and yet who quite deliberately chose to adopt that minor-key role.'

More than 600 persons requested interviews. 'I was absolutely swamped with unscheduled meetings and scores of appointments that kept me going from about seven am till eleven pm every day,' including press and television interviews. Many participants had arrived with authority from their countrymen to beg Graham to hold a crusade in their land, like the president of the Supreme Court of Cambodia, who had been converted from Buddhism by reading Billy Graham's book, *Peace with God*. The following spring, after the Khmer Rouge take-over, he and other prominent men were taken to a stadium and shot.

The Congress concluded with a great service of Holy Communion. The preacher before Communion was the Anglican bishop Festo Kivengere from Uganda, caught up in the realization that the Cross of Christ 'was the only possible answer to what we had been discussing.' His powerful sermon, and the distribution of the bread and wine to more than 4,000 people took far longer than intended. Graham, as he rose at last to give the closing address, 'The King Is Coming', felt himself somewhat an anticlimax, though no one shared that feeling. He was suffering much from an infected jaw and 'While I was speaking it was difficult to keep my mind on the message because of the pain. I was afraid to take a pain killer for fear I would not be alert.' Since it was already late in the morning he shortened his address.

He stressed the urgency to evangelize because of the certainty of Christ's return, and in calling for rededication and recommitment he did not hesitate to confess his own need. 'You know what God has been saying to you these past ten days, I know what He has convicted me of, and what I must do.' This public remark, which in fact referred to his private determination to cut out any lingering desire to play a political role in his own country, made a strong impression, especially on those from the Third World. 'Dr Graham confessing his own weaknesses – we thought we were the only ones that had problems like that. This was the most moving message for us!'

Closing his address, Billy touched on eight characteristics needed in a man or woman who would be an instrument that God can use. He ended: 'The problems with which we wrestle as we go back to our places of service are in many cases not intellectual. They lie deep down within the will.

Are we willing to deny self and to take up the Cross and follow the Lord? Are you willing? Am I willing? . . . The King is coming!'

Lausanne 1974 had become a date in Billy Graham's life comparable to 1949 and 1954. The Los Angeles campaign in the tent at the corner of Washington and Hill Streets in 1949 had made him a national figure. Five years later the Greater London Crusade of 1954 had brought him world fame. Twenty years after London, Lausanne showed him to be far more than an evangelist: he was a world Christian statesman, a catalyst who could bring individuals and movements to a fusion that set them on a new path for the glory of God.[1]

1. For a full account of the preparation, course and immediate aftermath of Lausanne, see *Evangelist to the World*, Chapters 15, 16 and 19.

Part Three
1977–

16

Into Eastern Europe

A remarkable six years began for Billy Graham in September 1977 with his breakthrough into an expanding ministry in eastern European communist countries. Simultaneously, more and more opportunities came in other parts of the world and in the United States. The period ended with his great conference of itinerant evangelists in the summer of 1983, which was not so much a climax as the opening of the next phase. His objectives were being fulfilled: to proclaim the gospel of Christ to as many people as possible; to build bridges of understanding between the peoples of the world; and to work for true peace between the nations.

On 3 September 1977, however, Billy, Ruth, Cliff and a small team met in a hotel in Vienna with considerable apprehension. They had been invited to Hungary. They knew that any hope of further ministry in the Socialist countries of Eastern Europe, and in the Soviet Union itself, hinged upon that one week's visit.[1]

For twenty years Billy had cherished a hope of preaching in Hungary. The invitation of 1977 came suddenly after five years of patient diplomacy by Walter Smyth and a Hungarian-American physician, surgeon and pastor, Alexander S. Haraszti of Atlanta; and as the result of the determination of a Hungarian free churchman, the late Sandor Palotay, a hunchback with a complex character who was president of the Council of Free Churches and unpopular with many Christians but devoted to their cause. He had recognized Graham's genius from afar, and risked position and career to bring him to Hungary.

Billy Graham was also at risk. The Socialist countries of eastern Europe formed the one large area of humanity, other

1. A fuller account is in *Evangelist to the World*, Chapter 24.

than mainland China, where he had never preached. He knew that some of his countrymen would accuse him of compromise with Communism, yet he could not refuse to minister to men and women because they lived under a different political ideology; most had no choice.

Billy's first main engagement in Hungary was to preach in the open air on Sunday afternoon in the grounds of the Baptist Youth camp above the Danube, sixteen miles north of Budapest. To conform with the State's rules governing religious liberty, the meeting had to be on church property, with no announcement in the press. Billy did not expect a big crowd and was astonished at the crush of humanity under the poplar and locust trees: the police estimated that 30,000 were present, all alerted by word of mouth and long distance telephone calls. A large number had been waiting since before dawn. Many came from other Warsaw Pact countries.

No restriction was placed on his message – otherwise he would not have come. The crowd warmed to his homely stories and responded to his plain preaching, impeccably translated by Haraszti. Hundreds put up a hand in response: a local estimate gave the figure as about 1,500. Many were young people from Christian homes, taking courage from the crowd to make an open commitment to Christ, which they knew could harm their careers; thus a Lutheran pastor's son, winner of four gold medals in the Olympic pentathlon, was quietly dropped from the team when it was known that he had consecrated his life at this meeting and would train to be a pastor.

Many Party officials and factory managers came out of curiosity but some with sincere interest. The Hungarian press reported Tahi briefly, putting the crowd figure low. As Billy travelled throughout Hungary in the next week, preaching to overflow crowds in small Baptist churches, the Hungarian people were kept from knowing much about it, though again and again Billy had evidence of the encouragement that his visit brought to believers, open and secret. If the country as a whole could not be reached, those who mattered in State and church were captivated. The secretary of state for church affairs, Imre Miklos, officially an atheist, became Billy's warm friend.

The two leading Protestant bishops, Kaldy of the

Lutherans and Bartha of the Reformed, had been openly critical of Billy Graham and had refused the use of their church buildings which would have held far more than those where the indoor meetings took place. Both bishops, out of courtesy, shared platforms with Billy. Talking to him informally and listening to his addresses swept away their mistaken belief that he was naive, narrow and unconcerned with the social role of the church. 'I was deeply impressed,' recalled Bartha a year later, 'by his warmth, his Christian spirit, his honesty, and his humility in saying, "I have come to learn." I took him to my heart.' Both recognized Billy's integrity; that he would not say one thing to their faces but another when he returned to the West. For one of the bishops, the visit was the beginning of a new flowering of his faith.

The coming of Billy Graham to Hungary proved to be a significant event in the improvement of relations between the atheist state and the Christian churches. It also restored the self-confidence of the smaller Protestant groups such as the Methodists and Baptists, who found new opportunities. It built a bridge between the Hungarian and American peoples, not least when the film made by the Billy Graham Association was shown across America on television. As the first of his films about Eastern Europe it had its weaknesses, yet taught Americans much about the life and religion of the land.

The Hungarian visit was a personal triumph for Billy, and made certain the opening of other socialist countries. And it gave him a new ministry in speaking to atheist high officials and Party members about the living Christ.

One year later came the ten day 'Evangelization of Billy Graham' in Poland, a country predominantly and vigorously Roman Catholic, yet ruled by atheists. After negotiations by the same team the invitation came from the Polish Baptist Union and the Polish Ecumenical Council which represents the non-Catholic minority. The remarkably skilful organization of the tour was done by the small Baptist denomination, especially its president, Michael Stankiewicz. Director Tadeuz Dusik of the state office for religious affairs (who became warm friends with Billy) was most helpful. The

Catholics opened their churches to Billy Graham in an unprecedented gesture: the trust between Stankiewicz and two key Catholic officials, Bishops Dabrowski and Misiolek, was a vital factor, but Cardinal Wojtyla of Kracow gave warmest support to the invitation. When Billy reached Kracow Wojtyla had gone to Rome to be elected Pope John Paul II on the very day on which Billy Graham left Poland.

Every meeting place was full for hours before the service. In Warsaw the main Lutheran, Reformed and Baptist churches were used, and the great Catholic church of All Saints, with its fine paintings and huge baroque altar below a painting of the resurrection and the glory of Christ. The Baptist choir stood in front of the altar, and the crowds stretched out of the church on to the green: this was not church property, yet the police did not disperse them.

Here, and in his whirlwind tour of five other cities, Billy preached in great simplicity: this, and his sincerity, reached priests and people, hungry for a deepening of their lives at a time of the growing economic and social crisis which erupted less than a year later.

At Katowice, the coal mining city which would be much in the headlines in the early days of Solidarity, the enormous modern cathedral of Christ the King was filled to capacity, with 13,000 people covering the red carpets in the aisles which converge on the altar, and out on to the terrace. They listened in total silence as Billy preached on the text from Galatians: 'God forbid that I should glory, save in the cross of our Lord Jesus Christ.' At Katowice, unlike most of the churches, a counselling area was available; those who made commitments to Christ went down into the crypt, with its shrine of the franciscan priest who gave his life for another man in Auschwitz. Here 2,000 persons were counselled. The Bishop of Katowice, Herbert Bednorz, had asked the Baptists: 'How many members do you have in Katowice?' 'Three hundred,' they replied. 'Then how will you fill my cathedral?' He was astonished and delighted at the great attendance, 'the greatest ecumenical event in the history of my diocese,' he said from the pulpit. He wrote to Billy two months later that the ecumenical meeting in the cathedral had deepened and strengthened the unity of Christians in his diocese, and that when he went to a conference of the bishops from all over Poland, 'your preaching was very positively estimated.'

The 'Evangelization of Billy Graham' greatly increased respect and understanding among the majority Catholics for the Baptists. Many Catholics joined the follow-up groups and learned to study the Bible, thus encouraging a new movement that was already gaining ground in Poland. Billy's visit induced an immediate marked increase in the sales of Bibles. Shortage of paper prevented the demand being met fully at first, but it was no passing phase: two years later, in the three months between November 1982 and January 1983 the Bible Society in Warsaw sold nearly 47,000 Bibles and more than 36,000 New Testaments.

If Billy Graham influenced Poland, Poland also influenced Billy Graham. It gave him more assurance, and encouragement and experience in helping Christians in the difficult circumstances of eastern Europe. It brought him more contacts and friendships towards his further ministry in socialistic countries. And it brought him the profound experience of the visit to Auschwitz.

He and Ruth had been briefed, back in Montreat, by a senior official of the United States government about the consequences of a nuclear war between the superpowers. The grim facts, expounded in accurate detail five years before the general public were given impressions by a television company, appalled the Grahams. Billy realized as never before that the human race could destroy itself in a matter of hours. 'Man's technology has leaped far ahead of his moral ability to control his technology. As I searched the Scriptures, my responsibilities dawned on me.' He determined to speak out.

He chose the visit to the Auschwitz concentration camp between Kracow and Katowice, preserved as a memorial, to make his first public statement on the need for nuclear disarmament by all nations: 'The very survival of human civilization is at stake . . . The present insanity of a global arms race, if continued, will lead inevitably to a conflagration so great that Auschwitz will seem a minor rehearsal.' In a widely reported speech he called on world leaders, whatever their ideology, to put national pride and power second to the survival of the human race, and called on all Christians to rededicate themselves 'to the Lord Jesus Christ, to the cause of peace, to reconciliation among all the races and nations of the world.'

He delivered his speech standing before the 'Wall of Death', where 20,000 prisoners were executed. He was almost in tears after being conducted round the gas chambers and the camp, with its vivid memorials of human suffering. The wall now had a cross, where visitors put flowers. Billy and Ruth had placed a wreath there and had knelt in prayer. Auschwitz drove deep into Billy's mind his growing concern for nuclear disarmament. He would urge it publicly and privately – not unilateral disarmament but the total destruction, by all nations, of nuclear, biological or chemical and laser weapons.

To preach true peace between nations and in the hearts of men would be part of his world ministry henceforth. The arms race became 'my number one social concern.'

In January 1981 Billy was back in Poland to receive an honorary degree in theology before proceeding to Hungary for another, shown on state television, and then to Rome for a private meeting with the Pope.

Meanwhile, in Poland 'The Evangelization of Billy Graham' continued to exert influence. 'Your ministry has exceeded all our expectations and imaginations,' wrote his interpreter, Zdzislaw Pawlik, who was also secretary of the ecumenical council. 'It was really a historic event in terms of uniting all Christians around the Word of God and giving new impetus to the life of individuals and congregations.' It had come at a strategic moment in Poland's history: the election of Pope John Paul II immediately after; the rise of Solidarity, the new freedoms; the period of martial law.

On 1 June 1983 the film of his 1978 tour, which had profoundly impressed America, was shown on Polish television, which had been barred to religious programmes at the time of his visit. Between four and five million Poles watched this film with its brilliant photography and clear message of the need for a simple faith in Christ, 'It can be regarded as a very important contribution,' commented Pawlik. 'It was received very well by the Polish people.'

Billy Graham, already evangelist to five continents, was now plainly evangelist to the world.

17

Tidal Wave

During the Metro Manila crusade of December 1977, the President of the Philippines broke precedent by giving a state dinner for the Grahams and the Team after one of the crusade meetings; no religious leader, not even Pope Paul VI or Pope John Paul II, received a similar honour. Thanking Billy for bringing 'the freshness of the spirit and the joy that comes from knowing God,' President Marcos continued: 'You come as a peacemaker, you come as one who has the same deep aspirations for the brotherhood of all humanity. And you seek, too, to lift up that miserable two-thirds of mankind who belong to the Third World, our world of abject poverty, ignorance, misery, our world desperately in need of God.'

The President's words were shortly to prove particularly apt. After a closing service when 150,000 people came to Ritzal Park, Billy flew from Manila to India. While the Filipino follow up committee were handling more than 22,000 inquirers, of whom 60 per cent were Roman Catholic, including a leading film star who became a renowned evangelist, Billy conducted 'Good News Festivals' in Calcutta and three other cities. But two weeks earlier a devastating cyclone and the worst tidal wave since 1864 had struck the coast of Andhra Pradesh in South India, causing 10,000 deaths, wiping out villages and inflicting untold loss and misery.

The President of India, receiving Graham in New Delhi, begged his help. As soon as Billy reached Hyderabad-Secunderabad, capital of the stricken state, he announced to the great crowd which attended the Good News Festival that his World Relief Fund would give $21,000 for rebuilding churches: the sum had been raised at the recent Cincinnati crusade. At Madras, the closing Festival of the tour, he left

Akbar Haqq to preach at one of the five services and flew in a plane chartered by the Team to the devastated area. The government provided a helicopter from the local airport.

As Billy landed he could see funeral pyres, and as he walked in the washed out fields and villages, where relief workers helped feed orphans and put up shelter, more bodies were recovered and he prayed over them. Survivors took his hands in theirs: 'Kill us or build us houses,' pleaded one, in a harrowing scene which was afterwards seen on film by millions.

Billy was escorted by the state minister of education, a devout Hindu who had been at his home in the immediate area on the night of the disaster. He had taken charge of relief. It was he who suggested that Billy Graham build in his own name an entire new village. The minister pointed out that Indians always pronounce the name as *Billy Gram*, and that the word for 'village' in Telegu, the local language, is *gram*. Billy agreed at once.

Other organizations were sending relief quickly but Billy's coming in person, and his grief and love, touched all India. Indians called him 'Angel of Mercy'.

On return to America he immediately raised money. The film of the festivals and of the cyclone disaster, shown on television, brought in $100,000. Meanwhile the Team set up the Andhra Pradesh Christian Relief and Rehabilitation committee, headed by the two co-chairmen of the festival: the Roman Catholic Archbishop of Hyderabad and a leading Baptist, Ch. Devananda Rao, who was minister of tourism in the state cabinet, and had come with Billy to the scene of the disaster. Plans for the new model township were drawn quickly. The state government gave nearly a quarter of the cost of the houses; the Billy Graham Association raised more than three quarters, and the cost of the church and the water tower. On April 21, 1978, only six months after the tidal wave, Archbishop Arulappa dedicated the foundation stone of Billy Graham Naga.

It was not, therefore, the crowds at the festivals, nor the 12,841 recorded decisions, nor (in the words of the Bishop in Madras) the 'great source of blessing to the entire Indian church,' which made the true significance of the Indian visit of December 1977; but the founding of Billy Graham Naga as a spontaneous gesture of Christian compassion.

Wherever he was, Billy Graham had never passed by on the other side. In younger days his preaching had been affected by reaction to the heresy of a 'social gospel'; Biblically based Christians had tended to forget the strong social conscience which had been one of the glories of the evangelical revival. As the years passed, Billy had done much to correct the balance among his contemporaries, while avoiding identification with particular political or social solutions to world or national problems. During the 1970s he channelled much money to famine and disaster relief, as well as to education in the Third World, and his sponsorship of Lausanne had led to theological rethinking on the relationship between evangelism and social action.

Thus his response, and the Team's, to the Indian cyclone disaster was typical, and they took close interest in the progress of Billy Graham Naga. The President of India promised to come for the inauguration of the completed township if Billy came too, but this did not prove possible.

Instead Franklin Graham, now president of World Medical Missions and of Samaritan's Purse, represented his father. On a hot Sunday, 29 June 1980, two years and nine months after the night of terror and grief, Franklin, Walter Smyth and others from the Team were met by the villagers, 'bubbling with joy'. Two hundred and eighty-five new houses were already occupied by survivors of the disaster, forming a mixed community of Catholics, Protestants and non-Christians. They crowded happily round, with the local leaders of church and state, as Franklin dedicated Billy Graham Naga and its new church of St John the Baptist.

By his World Emergency Fund Billy and the Team continued to do 'all we can to help people on every continent, especially when disaster strikes. For example,' he told the students at Harvard in 1982, 'our organization has helped build hospitals in such diverse places as Zaire, Jordan, Israel, India. We've sent plane after plane load of medical supplies and food supplies to various areas of the world where there were refugees. We helped support a boat picking up the boat people in the South China Seas. And my son worked on that

135

boat. And I could cite scores of incidents that have come about as a result of the growing responsibility we feel toward the oppressed and the needy in the world.

'In addition, I've tried to use privately what little influence I may have had with those in high places to do something on a governmental level: not just to give relief, but to work toward changes. And, on occasion, have succeeded.

'My pilgrimage has also let me to call for morality and ethics in government. During our history, we've gone through many traumatic periods, in which we almost lost confidence in all forms of government. But the problem was not necessarily the form of government, but the ambitions and moral blindness of some of those in power. The kind of government any nation has will be determined by the kind of ethics and morality which underlie the political structure. But it also will depend on the moral integrity we demand of those in leadership. Government will never be better than the men and women who have given their lives to it.

'And they will never be better than the world and life-view they accept, and on which they operate. Either the law of love will prevail – or the law of hatred, violence, and dishonesty will prevail.'

18

Sydney 1979

The Archbishop of Sydney, Sir Marcus Loane, was attending a missionary conference in the mountains of West Irian in 1975. He went for a hike by himself. While walking he reflected that 1979 would be the twentieth anniversary of the crusade of 1959, and that two years later he was due to retire. On return to New South Wales he wrote on 29 July 1975 to Billy Graham: 'I long to see a fresh and mighty spiritual impact on our city and country. Under God, I believe that you are the man to head up this task.'

The Archbishop was certain the crusade must not be short; when Billy had returned for ten days in 1968 many had come forward and joined the churches but the obvious impact had been small. Loane therefore made three weeks (four Sundays) a condition. He showed the letter to Bishop Jack Dain, still closely in touch with Graham since Lausanne. Dain commented that such an invitation was hardly worth its stamp, for Billy had not taken a three week crusade for years, nor had he given a firm date so far ahead. Walter Smyth walked in before the letter was mailed, and expressed his gratitude to Loane but could offer no assurance of acceptance.

Billy replied on 12 August that if ever he returned to Sydney he would like to come while Marcus Loane was Archbishop, and that he favoured three weeks. 'However, keep in mind that I will be sixty years old and will not have near the physical vigor and stamina that I had in 1959 . . . It would be difficult for me to describe how much large stadium evangelistic meetings take out of me physically now. By God's grace I can still do it—but I have to limit myself to the evening meetings.'

Late that year the Archbishop brought together the heads and prominent ministers of the other denominations. After a small hesitation because the Archbishop had approached

Graham before consulting them, they gave unanimous support: 'there will be an enormous volume of goodwill and prayer from the beginning,' Graham was assured. He accepted, in January 1976, and preparation began.

The venue of 1959, the Royal Agricultural Showground, would not be available. The only site of sufficient size was Randwick racecourse, which would unexpectedly be free (except for one meeting which the Jockey Club transferred) because of a court case two years before the crusade. Geographically Randwick was the wrong side of the city from the new areas of expansion. Moreover the shape of a racecourse, despite expert adaptation, would prevent the sense of crowd which a stadium or the Showground gives; but it was specially suitable for interpretation to the ethnic minorities, grown much larger.

With three years to go preparations were perhaps more thorough and deeper than any previous crusade throughout the world; all the lessons of the past thirty years were assimilated and adapted to reach a city which had changed much in population, style and skyline since 1959. Jack Dain became chairman. As none of the American Team was available, Billy and Walter chose the Australian Barry Berryman, head of the Association's office in Sydney, to be crusade director, the first time that a national had directed a Billy Graham crusade, but an inspired choice. Of the twenty-six chairmen of committees, two were converts of '59, one as a schoolboy, the other as a young professional man who had not been a churchgoer. Many committee men and women were also converts.

The diocese of Sydney fashioned its programme to prepare and follow up the crusade. As the diocesan director of evangelism said, they took the opportunity 'to do everything we had ever dreamed of doing, under the guise of getting ready for Billy Graham.' Canon John Chapman added that only Billy could have brought the Protestant denominations of Sydney (apart from a very few individual churches) to work together so closely and effectively. The Roman Catholics did not co-operate, but did not oppose.

By late April 1979, when Billy and Ruth took the plane for Australia, Sydney had been saturated with prayer because prayer groups had spread like wildfire. Counsellors were trained. Five thousand nurture groups were ready to receive those who came forward. There had been widespread 'dialogue evangelism', and training to reach the population of high rise blocks. The churches had set so much going that all would have been worthwhile, they felt, even had Billy dropped dead.

He arrived in Sydney ten days before the Crusade's opening, and at once won the ear of the city through the friendly welcome of the press. He had met privately in New York, six weeks earlier, an Australian newspaper magnate for a most constructive discussion. At the airport press conference Billy's sincerity and humility won the immediate support of hard pressmen, who then followed the lead of one of them, Alan Gill of *Sydney Morning Herald,* a strong Christian.

Billy was soon on television. In 1959 he had needed to overcome the fear of Australians that he was either a 'wowser' or a hypocrite. In 1979 they already admired and accepted him as 'fair dinkum', but the television chat shows gave him opportunity to put the Gospel into living rooms in a relaxed yet decisive way: Sydney loved him for his answers to a star interviewer's problems with kangaroos in the Ark; even more effective were Billy's clear replies to the celebrated Mike Willesee, who asked whether Billy were a saint; and the final moments of David Frost's show when Frost suddenly asked him to close the programme with prayer.

Billy also addressed a large lunchtime audience of leading businessmen, many of whom were not churchgoers. Billy held them spellbound. One elderly magnate called it 'one of the finest hours I have spent in my lifetime listening to him.' Ruth Graham, on another day, spoke equally effectively to the women of Sydney, filling the new Opera house beside the harbour.

Spring weather in Sydney is usually mild and mainly dry. Instead it turned cold and wet. On the evening that Randwick racecourse was handed to the crusade executive to be adapted, the architect and his assistant drove in from opposite sides of Sydney through rain, only to find

Randwick strangely dry until the coffee break at midnight: the women's prayer groups had prayed.

The crusade opened in rain. Evening after evening the rain and wind made the racecourse no pleasant place to attend a service in the open. The weather reduced the crowds but could not dampen the enthusiasm of the thousands who came as a result of Operation Andrew. Those who were not in the covered stands sat on specially provided plastic sacks.

One evening, during a violent thunderstorm, lightning knocked out the sound system shortly before it was due to be turned on, after the choir rehearsal. The Australian sound crew did all they could to salvage enough equipment to reach the crowd, smaller than usual because of the storm, but without success. Bill Fasig, the Team member at the control, telephoned Cliff Barrows on the platform. Cliff replied: 'I will keep the choir rehearsing, and you pray.' The contractor said to Fasig: 'You might as well. We have done everything else!'

The sound came on exactly as the service was due to start. The contractor was astounded. 'What did you do?' he asked. 'I prayed,' replied Fasig.

Billy was deeply grateful for the way the committee and the hundreds of crusade volunteers 'faced the overwhelming problems of rain, weather, and even the venue itself. You did it with courage and faith and without complaining. You took it all as from the Lord. This was an inspiration and a blessing to all of us.'

The lower attendance affected finance. The budget had not been met before the crusade began, as the finance committee had hoped. Therefore an offertory appeal was made each evening, directed solely to Christians in the audience, and emphasizing that Billy and the Team received no remuneration for their services, and that the money would be spent in Australia. After a week and a half the budget was still not met. Billy offered to make the offertory appeal himself.

The finance committee and its chairman, Neville Malone, a senior accountant in the oil industry, declined: only Australians should appeal to Australians for money. With the shortfall now serious, Billy renewed his offer, provided the crusade's inner executive agreed unanimously.

Malone held out alone, and Billy stayed silent. Malone and his friends and prayer partners continued to pray earnestly, and suddenly the money began to come, but the budget needed to be increased, and Bishop Dain again urged that Billy be allowed to speak. Malone again declined. Malone spoke before the offertory on the last night but one, in a spiritual, unemotional and rather original way that impressed Billy so much that he took Malone's notes. On the last night Dain made a low key request to Christians that they give sacrificially. Many non-churchgoers gave too.

The budget was met. Money poured in after the crusade. The big surplus would have been put to making the film of the crusade, *A Time for Decision*, had not a member of the finance committee already paid for it from his pocket.

The whole experience profoundly influenced Malone's own giving. Later he left industry to serve as treasurer of the diocese.

Meanwhile, despite the rain and the wind, inquirers were coming forward. Billy preached more slowly than in 1959, and older Australians found the content deeper and more expository, the delivery less melodramatic yet equally powerful and clear, especially to the young. The percentage of inquirers stayed almost constant. The Archbishop, whose unbroken attendance emphasized to Sydney the crusade's importance, said in a speech six months later: 'Such a crusade is a phenomenon for which one can hardly account on a human level. The best part of Billy Graham by the grace of God is Billy Graham: a man whose face and voice have those qualities of unaffected humility and total sincerity. It will never cease to amaze when one recalls the invitation and response at each meeting; almost the same words for the same appeal, and the instant, silent flood of men and women surging quietly forward from every corner and every grandstand.'

On the night of the worst weather a federal cabinet minister's wife slushed through the mud: her testimony was very effective to women's groups in the months to come. Another night came an elderly and distinguished paedo-physician, whose witness in the short remaining years of his life, and his funeral, were long remembered.

Most of those who came forward were ordinary citizens, many of them young. One night a member of the crusade executive, exhausted, was tempted to give up. Then a fellow member said: 'My church had a hundred referrals last week.' The news was like a shot in the arm: the hard work was worthwhile for the fresh life pouring into the churches.

In the last week the weather cleared and numbers rose sharply. Billy, meanwhile, rather to his own surprise, felt fitter than when he had begun. And the crusade was reaching right across Australia through videos and landlines, to hospitals, churches, mission stations in the outback, and even to households where neighbours would be invited. Twenty-nine out of the thirty-six television stations of Australia carried some of the meetings.

At Sydney itself in the three week crusade 21,331 people went forward as inquirers, compared with the 56,780 in the four weeks of 1959. But Sydney churches were more ready and able to garner the fruit. An incomplete survey a year later suggested that the influence might even be deeper than 1959, for it showed that 63 per cent of inquirers were still regularly attending the church to which they had been referred, and that 36 per cent of the inquirers had not previously been churchgoers. The survey also showed that the major wastage occurred immediately after the crusade. Of those who joined nurture classes or churches, few failed to become settled, growing Christians; and to judge from crusades elsewhere, such as at Rio in 1974, many of those who did not come forward, or who came but did not join a church, would find no happiness until they responded to Christ, perhaps years later.

Six months after the crusade the Archbishop of Sydney declared to his diocesan synod: 'I would like to think that Sydney has been stirred and touched to its depths by a mighty movement of the Spirit of God and that thousands of its people will prove to have experienced a radical and permanent change in their lives.'

And in 1981, a few months before his retirement, Sir Marcus reflected on the result of his walk in West Irian all those years before: 'The crusade did not make the break-through or the impact on the city at large in the way that one would have hoped, but I would say without reservation that it was a source of very great blessing to the churches, among churchpeople and for those whom church people were personally responsible for bringing.'

19

Great Steps Forward

On 13 September 1980 many evangelical leaders and other guests, including George Bush, soon to be elected Vice President of the United States, came together for the dedication of a fine new building in the Colonial style on the campus of Wheaton College: the Billy Graham Center.

For nearly thirty years Graham had considered founding an educational institution. At one time he had thoroughly investigated the possibility of creating a new university, but every project was laid aside because it might deflect him from his primary task of evangelism. At length, in the later 1970s, he found his answer. In September 1977 he turned the first sod on the site of a warehouse which Wheaton, his *alma mater*, had cleared away on donating the land. The building rose fast. Billy appointed a Team member to raise funds, and gave to the Center the royalties of his next book to be published; as this was *Angels*, which became a runaway best seller and topped the American non-fiction list for weeks, the Center's finance had a good start.

The 'Billy Graham Center at Wheaton College' soon established itself as an aid to Christian enterprise and thought, to the understanding of the past and to planning for the future. Associated with the Wheaton Graduate School it helps prepare future leaders from all over the world, intellectually and spiritually. It organizes courses and conferences to think through the problems and possibilities confronting the Church. The Library provides an impetus to the study of evangelism and missions through the ages and in the contemporary world. The Archives not only bring together in expert hands the vast and growing mass of papers relating to the Billy Graham crusades, and Graham's life and ministry; they are a repository for the manuscripts of American evangelists and thus an important centre of research.

And there is the Museum. During the building of the Center Billy became concerned that the Museum might be a glorification of himself. He wanted to scrap it. He was dissuaded, and the finished product delighted him. Designed by a sensitive expert, it provides the visitor with 'a walk through the Gospel', setting American revivals and the Billy Graham crusades into the context of church history from earliest times. and featuring the varied ways in which the Christian message reaches the contemporary world.

'The Museum deeply moved me and filled me with silence, wonder and tears,' wrote one of the distinguished guests at the dedication. 'I wanted at the end to be alone with Jesus for as long a time as He would please to grant me.'

Immediately after the dedication Billy left for Japan. A crusade in Tokyo and three other cities, with Leighton Ford preaching at two more, had been prepared, in much prayer, with outstanding thoroughness.

Billy had briefed himself fully about this highly populated industrial nation with a strongly traditional culture. The stranglehold of tradition and of the ancient religions was loosening; the young were open to other influences, though not to Marxism, which had little appeal to Japanese. Christianity had been preached freely for more than a hundred years, yet only one per cent of the people were Christians. At a dinner before Billy's Osaka crusade the governor of the province asked why so few in Japan believed the Christian gospel. He answered his own question in a memorable phrase: 'Perhaps, because it has not been made clear.'

Billy Graham had already helped to make it clear. Thirteen years earlier, in 1967, he had held a Tokyo crusade which had proved to be a milestone in Japanese history, turning the eyes of an inward looking church to the urgency of the need to reach the nation. Nineteen sixty-seven had done much to tip the balance away from the negative liberalism which had dominated the united church (of the larger denominations) since before the Second World War.

Nineteen eighty carried this process a great step further. In origin and preparation the crusade was essentially Japanese.

145

Tensions – between local committees and the national, between the older and the younger leaders, between nationals and the American advisory team under Henry Holley – had been resolved by graciousness and a shared determination that nothing should weaken the thrust of the Gospel.

Billy arrived in the first days of October 1980. After a press conference in Tokyo, where every enterprise should begin, he flew south to Okinawa. There, and in each city afterwards, the crusade surprised even those with most faith. Japan was startled by the great numbers which gathered, and because numbers mean much to the Japanese, they awarded a new respect to Christianity, which suddenly became more visible. In the months and years afterwards this helped to make the people more open to the message which Christians preached.

Billy knew that when he gave the invitation to receive Christ, many might come forward without fully understanding what a decision would cost to their future lives. He therefore made the invitation tough. As in Korea seven years earlier he emphasized that they should get out of their seats only if they would forsake all other gods. 'I thought no one would respond,' wrote Billy from Tokyo, 'but last night we had over 2,000. In Fukuoka, which has only 1,000 Christians, it poured torrential rain and yet we had from 15–17,000 people at each service sitting in the open, and hundreds responding to the appeal (in water that sometimes went over their shoe tops). I am not a church historian enough to evaluate what is happening, but I believe that Japan may be on the verge of a Christian revival.'

In Tokyo, after the baseball stadium had overflowed with people and many had streamed forward to be counselled, the Japanese pastors were 'shouting happy' at all that had happened. Their follow up system had gone smoothly into action. The next years brought many new members to the churches; hundreds of other inquirers slipped out of sight but the pastors were not discouraged, knowing that in Japan a conversion could be a very slow process.

Japan was not likely to see a spectacular turning to Christ as in Korea, but city-wide evangelism became easier because the barriers between churches had dropped for Billy Graham. The crusade had strengthened the faith and courage of the small minority of Japanese who were Christians, and their determination to make Christ's message clear to their friends.

Six months after the crusade Walter Smyth was back in Japan to meet representatives from every crusade city. 'It was one of the most thrilling evenings I have ever spent,' for they reminded him that the average Japanese Protestant church had less than fifty members, then told him of church after church which had already baptized thirty or forty people.

Yet the crusade had been only a step. Most of their countrymen remained without Christ. The Japanese longed that Billy Graham should return in the mid-1980s, for they held that he was 'God's man for this age'.

Several Osaka pastors once discussed why Billy could reach the Japanese so decisively. 'Billy Graham is a very humble person,' said one, 'and he loves the heart of common people. He knows the condition of the soul and applies the Gospel to them.' Another made two points: 'One, his emphasis is on prayer. He asked how many people pray: prayer moves the power of God. Another point, his Gospel is very simple. Many years ago Billy Graham came to St Paul University in Tokyo. He pointed out that we should preach to people so that even a 12-year-old boy could understand.'

And the third pastor said that Billy Graham 'has two faces. One face: his authority when on the platform. Short sentences and strong convictions. He gave us his message. He's a very authoritative person on the platform. The other face: when we speak together around the table he's just like a servant, a very humble person. He has a heart to listen to other people's opinions.'

From East to West: in the spring of 1981 Billy went to Mexico and the story could not have been more different from Japan's.

'The National Mexican Congress with Billy Graham' (for historical reasons the word 'crusade' could not be used) was planned in two halves: the first in Mexico City and the second at Villahermosa, capital of the state of Tabasco. The constitution of Mexico prohibits large public religious meetings except on church property. This rule was not broken for the Pope, though most Mexicans are nominally Catholics, and the sole exception remained a Billy Graham rally in the Arena Mexico in 1958. Hopes of inviting Billy back for a longer visit had foundered because of this problem.

During 1980, however, the congress committee secured a verbal promise of the Inde-Olympico stadium: the promise was never put in writing but given with enough assurance to justify going ahead. The Roman Catholic hierarchy, unlike their brethren in the Philippines, opposed the congress, though not openly until after it was over, when they declared Billy Graham a 'non-Christian'.

In Mexico City the committee planned haphazardly. Charles Ward of the Team, with his long experience of Latin America, had an uphill task as director. Villahermosa, was a contrast. Evangelicals had long flourished in the city and upstate, and Ward and his assistants found strong local leadership and overflowing zeal. When Bob Williams and Blair Carlson toured the state they were 'attracted to the loving spirit of the people. They welcomed us with open arms, served gourmet meals of the native Indian food, sat on the edge of their wooden benches, or stood for two hours of counsellor training. During the choir rehearsals we were amazed to hear beautiful harmony from the lips of these simple people. In a little town near the Guatemalan border over 200 people packed into the little Presbyterian church. What a glow on their faces! They were preparing and praying for the upcoming congress as if it were the event of the century.'

Another place was cut off by a flash flood and the Americans arrived two hours late after walking through the mud. The people were waiting with unabated enthusiasm.

In January 1981, six weeks before the congress was due, the Inde-Olympic stadium was suddenly closed down for the next few months because of a government official's speculation and the resulting law suits. The congress could obtain no alternative site until the evangelicals threatened to 'take to the streets'; the government held out to the last minute, then allowed the use of the much smaller Arena Mexico where Billy had preached in 1958. All the printed publicity was now worthless.

The Arena proved to be much too small for the tens of thousands who turned up to hear Billy. Many from up-country arrived too late and hammered on doors which had been closed by the authorities when the crowd exceeded the capacity and the fire safety point was reached. Others went in error to the original site.

Committee and Team alike were amazed by the response when Billy gave the invitation. The nominally Catholic but largely secularized Mexicans hungered for the Gospel. Down at Villahermosa where an 8,000 seat baseball stadium had at least 35,000 people in it every night, the response was over-whelming. 'Literally thousands,' wrote Ward, 'surrounded the platform. The counsellors could not begin to cope with the numbers, so we passed out our "Commitment to Christ" folder and a decision card for the people themselves to fill out.' Fortunately the follow up had been well planned.

For the first time in Mexican history the evangelical (i.e. Protestant) Church became national news. The press at Mexico City were cool at first, then warm and excited. At Villahermosa the press gave unstinted support; likewise the secular authorities.

Evangelicals had been barred from preaching on television, but Billy was invited to appear on several chat shows; in answer to questions he put across the Gospel freely and plainly. He visited the President of Mexico and opened many doors in high places which had been shut against evangelicals. Meanwhile a School of Evangelism in Mexico City, organized to coincide with the congress, brought together more than 1,400 ministers and lay persons, from all over Mexico and neighbouring countries, and made great impact on their lives. Billy described it as 'one of the best we have seen around the world.'

Billy's ten nights of preaching (seven in Mexico City and three in Villahermosa) opened a new chapter for Mexico.

20

Moscow 1982

At the end of February 1982 Billy Graham went to Blackpool in the north of England for a conference address and a two day crusade. The friendly crowds, and the hundreds who came forward, were unaware that he was wrestling with one of the most difficult decisions of his life: whether to accept a specific invitation to Moscow.

Five years earlier when he was in Hungary, Baptists from Moscow headed by Alexei Bychkov, general secretary of the All Union Council of Evangelical Christians Baptists, had brought a general invitation. Even before the visit to Poland high level negotiations had begun between the Billy Graham Team, represented by Walter Smyth, Alexander Haraszti and John Akers, and the Soviet authorities who, being Marxist-Leninists committed to atheism. As with all diplomacy, the details cannot be made public for many years. Soviet officials knew that Graham wished to work alongside the churches registered by the state, but he made plain at a very early stage his concern about the restrictions on religious freedom, and for prisoners of conscience.

Graham was aware that before the Communists took power in 1917 the Russian Orthodox Church and the Tsarist state had restricted and had oppressed the Baptists and other nonconformists. Lenin, though an atheist, had allowed these a toleration for a few years in the 1920s, which had led to great growth, while the Orthodox in their turn were grievously oppressed. Following the death of Lenin and the rise of Stalin, all Christians in Russia went through the fire of persecution until a measure of freedom was restored during the Second World War as a tribute to their patriotism.

Billy Graham had visited Moscow as a tourist in 1959. Since that time he had been keenly interested in the great movement to Christianity among Soviet peoples, and the continued discrimination and varying pressures by agents of the Soviet state, particularly during the new wave of persecution under Khrushchev from 1959 until his fall in 1964. Graham learned from a reliable count by a Western expert that some 20,000 places of worship, including those of Muslims and Buddhists, were officially registered in the Soviet Union: a small figure compared with Britain or the United States. Many others were unregistered and therefore unrecognized by law. He knew that by 1980 Christians totalled about 60 million, so that with 50 million Moslems and 3½ million Jews the believers in one God could be estimated at well over 100 million out of a total population of 271 million. Believers vastly outnumbered actual members of the Communist Party (official reckoning, nearly 18 million) who controlled their lives.

The Graham Team's negotiations in Moscow and with the Soviet Embassy in Washington led to a provisional confidential understanding that he should make a preaching visit to churches in several cities throughout the Soviet Union in September 1979. This was postponed when east-west relations deteriorated after Afghanistan in December 1978. Over two years later Haraszti learned that Graham was one of the leaders of Christian and non-Christian religions whom the Orthodox Patriarch of Moscow and All Russia, Pimen, contemplated inviting in May 1982 to address a 'World Conference: Religious Workers for saving the Sacred Gift of Life from Nuclear Catastrophe'.

The first direct contact between the Billy Graham Team and the Russian Orthodox Church came in October 1981 at Geneva, when Alexander Haraszti met Father Vitaly Borovoy, the Patriarchate's chief liaison officer with the World Council of Churches. It was made clear to Borovoy that Graham, if he came, must be allowed to preach in the Moscow Baptist church and in an Orthodox church, possibly the Patriarchal cathedral. Haraszti then went back to Moscow (one of eight visits which he made in twelve months) and was introduced to Metropolitan Philaret of Minsk and Belorussia, chairman of the external affairs department of the Moscow Patriarchate, for detailed discussions. Philaret's sympathetic understanding was important.

151

The decision to accept or decline the Patriarch's invitation could not be easy. The Orthodox Church had come into deep spirituality through the deprivations and the persecutions of the past, yet the leadership kept in step with the state; the West expected the conference to be propaganda for the Soviet peace movement. Graham emphasized to Moscow that his deep concern for nuclear disarmament did not make him a unilateralist, and that he would come as an observer, not a participant; he would not therefore sign the conference final statement. He also insisted that he must, as an evangelist, preach the Gospel in Moscow without any restrictions on his message: a desire endorsed by Orthodox, Baptists and government officials.

As Haraszti, in close contact with Smyth and Akers, went back and forth from Russia, Billy conveyed his determination to speak publicly on the issue of human rights, but as a guest he would not utter denunciations: these might win approval in the West but extinguish future ministry in the eastern bloc. Moreover he had taken to heart some advice from Vatican sources, that in Eastern Europe you can achieve much if you do not shout it from the house tops.

He also insisted that he must visit the Siberian Pentecostals who had been in the American Embassy since June 1977, hoping to be allowed to emigrate. He urged that the issue be resolved before he came, but if not, he must visit them. The Soviet authorities were surprised that he cared about the 'Siberian Seven' (considered to be law breakers), but finally agreed with reluctance to a private, pastoral visit.

On 5 February 1982 Patriarch Pimen issued the formal invitation, the Baptists added theirs, and Haraszti carried them back to America. He presented the letter to Billy Graham on Sunday 14 February at the Essex House Hotel in New York, where Billy had brought a few close associates to discuss and pray about his answer. If he went to Moscow it would pave the way to a longer visit, because churchmen and state officials would come to know him and he would learn much; it would help the churches by enhancing their importance in the eyes of the secular rulers, who would be impressed that their churchmen could secure such a world famous figure. It would open the door to eastern European countries who waited on Moscow before inviting Graham. It would provide opportunity to give his testimony to Christ and preach the gospel in high places of an atheist state, and before leaders of non-Christian religions.

The pitfalls were equally plain, and one or two of the Billy Graham Team did not want him to go, fearing he would be used. In the next ten days he spoke with family and colleagues and experts. The State Department and the White House had been consulted already. 'I discussed the advisability of my going with former President Nixon and former Secretary of State Henry Kissinger, both longtime personal friends. Mr Nixon told me: "There is a great risk, but I believe that for the sake of the message you preach, the risk is worth it." ' To refuse Moscow, however, would end for ever the hope of public ministry in the Soviet Union.

Billy reached England and Blackpool still undecided, though working on a formal letter of acceptance. He continued to agonize and pray and to discuss. During each of the three days at Blackpool his mind was dominated by the pros and cons of going to Moscow, yet when he mounted the podium to preach he could shut it right out; vigour flowed in, and he preached as if he had carried no burden all day except for the people before him.

The more Billy prayed and deliberated, the more sure he became that God had opened this door. He must go through it whatever the personal cost. But the decision once made did not flood his soul with peace.

When his acceptance was announced the criticism began; he would be a pawn; he was naïve; he would throw a cloak of respectability over the Kremlin's religious policies. The American press reported, wrongly, that the President had asked him to cancel his acceptance. The Siberian six called upon him to announce that he would not go if they still had not received their exit visas; but Graham already knew that the Kremlin would be unmoved by the gesture. The West might applaud but the Soviet churches would be the losers. He refused to attempt a short term victory at the price of a long term defeat.

Billy Graham reached Moscow on the evening of Friday 7

May. He could not arrive physically refreshed, for he was in the middle of the long scheduled series of university lectures and public crusades in New England. He was projected at once into five and a half days of interviews, services, meetings, tours and functions, backed by that immense hospitality which is typically Russian. At his age of sixty-three and a half it seemed the most demanding schedule he had ever known.

Warm friendships sprang up between Billy and Pastor Bychkov of the Baptists and Metropolitan Philaret of the Orthodox, friendships which helped closer relations and respect between the churches.

Billy also met men of importance in the Kremlin, the most senior being the chairman of the Foreign Relations Committee, Boris Ponomarev, who also was a secretary of the Communist Party; he had held office in Government and party since Stalin's day and was a candidate member of the Politburo, and was to retain his position after the death of Brezhnev. The two talked entirely alone for over an hour. Neither revealed details but, as Billy said later, at every interview 'I took the liberty of telling about Jesus Christ and what He means to me and how anyone can find Him.' 'It was graciously done,' commented an aide who was present at other interviews, 'but always very directly. And Billy comes across so well at private meetings.'

Billy knew that the rigid hold of Marxist-Leninist doctrine kept these men ignorant of Christianity and supposing that the things of the Spirit were delusions, to be explained by political or economic circumstances; yet each, like every human soul, had a hunger for God, however suppressed. Billy knew too of the widespread disappointment at the lack of idealism in Communist societies, the desire for answers that have eluded them.

He always raised the question of the Siberian six and of believers who were in prison: he had a list of about 150 in his hand. These matters were discussed frankly.

On the Saturday evening Billy was taken to three Orthodox Churches. The faithful pour into the few churches on a Saturday evening to prepare themselves for Sunday. In the world capital of atheism this weekday worship never fails to

154

move a western Christian. Billy commented to one of the newsmen who pressed after him everywhere that such a sight would not be seen on a Saturday night in Charlotte, North Carolina (where most of the numerous churches are not normally used on Saturday night.) He was astounded afterwards to find himself reported in the American press as saying that he found more religion in Moscow than in Charlotte.

That night came the first hitch. The Team were informed that Graham's preaching at the Baptist church, scheduled for 5 p.m. on Sunday, had been switched to 8 a.m., squeezed in before the Orthodox Divine Liturgy at 10.00 a.m. This washed out any unhurried meeting with the Baptists after service, while many of those coming from far would arrive too late.

The Baptists had begged the Graham Team to keep the 5 p.m. time confidential, lest too great a crowd should seek to attend. Unfortunately, under pressure of the media in America, the time had been mentioned earlier and The Voice of America and the B.B.C. had broadcast it to the Soviet Union. State authorities became alarmed at the prospect of half Moscow converging on the 2,000 seat Baptist church and ordered the change.

Next morning the police (peoples' militia) set up barriers and allowed only ticket holders to enter the Baptist church but they did not break up the overflow crowds in the narrow street. Nor did the police stop them singing hymns, although this is forbidden by law outside church property; next day The Times in London had a headline: 'Graham breaks new ground in Moscow.' He broke new ground in another way too, when the controlled Soviet media reported his activities. No previous religious visitor (apart from proponents of Soviet 'peace' movements) had been noticed. Christianity was barred from newspapers or television except as a target for ridicule or atheist propaganda, and Christians were therefore most excited to find Pravda reporting with respect the activities of an evangelist: his words brought Christianity to the masses.

Inside the Baptist 'prayer house' (as Protestant churches are called in Russia) the capacity attendance included

155

perhaps two thirds who were Moscow Baptists and their guests, some from the farthest republics of the Soviet Union. Perhaps a third were western and Soviet pressmen – and security personnel, so that at least some atheists were present. During Graham's sermon from *John* 5 a girl let down a banner for a few seconds from the left balcony; its English was fully plain to the Western press: 'We have 150 in prison', but Billy was involved in his preaching and was not looking in that direction at the time.

The joyful service ran overtime, as Russian services tend to, and Billy's Baptist hosts were nervous that he would be rudely late for the Divine Liturgy at the Patriarchal Cathedral, for a distinguished guest, who was to give greetings and a brief Biblican exposition, would show discourtesy to the Russian and foreign dignitaries if he were excessively late. The Baptists bundled him out of a side door into the car and away.

As he was getting into the car a newsman shouted, 'There's a large crowd waiting several blocks away to greet you.' Graham asked the driver if he would stop immediately. His escort (including a Baptist clergyman) said, 'There is absolutely no time because we are now twenty minutes late where you are expected at the Cathedral.' Graham, not realizing the significance of the crowd behind the barriers that wanted to greet him, but realizing the importance of speaking in one of Moscow's great Orthodox Cathedrals, agreed. He changed clothes in the car, and put on his robe and hood.

Waves of disappointment touched many a home in Moscow and beyond, especially among Christians who had travelled from far for a glimpse and to greet him.

At the cathedral of the Epiphany the matchless singing of the choirs and the intoning of the ancient liturgy by richly vested priests continued for two hours, followed by greetings. Then Billy Graham was invited to stand before the great golden screen or *ikonostasis* beside Patriarch Pimen. Nearby stood the Patriarchs of Alexandria, of Romania and Bulgaria, and many metropolitans and bishops.

Billy thanked Patriarch Pimen. On this Victory Day (May 9) he spoke of the sacrifice of the millions in the war and then of Christ's sacrifice. 'You can be partakers of his resurrection,' he continued. The interpreter had no amplifier. There were cries of 'Louder! Louder!' The next sentences therefore rang out through the church: 'This Jesus is the perfect atonement for our sins. He is standing at the right hand of glory and will return victorious.'

The conference for 'Saving the Sacred Gift of Life from Nuclear Catastrophe' opened next day. When Billy's turn came he delivered a long, far ranging speech on the Christian Faith and Peace in a Nuclear Age. Jewish, Buddhist, Hindu and Moslem leaders heard him. Many atheists from Soviet government circles were present, and his reasoned but uncompromising exposition of the Biblical answer to world problems and to the nuclear threat was possibly the most resounding public affirmation of the Christian gospel to be heard in Moscow outside a church for more than sixty years. Many of his statements ran contrary to Moscow's accepted thinking, for he emphasized the value and dignity of the individual, and that God is the Lord of history, and that 'lasting peace will only come when the Kingdom of God prevails. The basic issue that faces us today is not merely political, social, economic, or even moral or humanitarian. The deepest problems of the human race are spiritual. They are rooted in man's refusal to seek God's way for his life. The problem is the human heart, which God alone can change.'

One section was entirely devoted to human rights and religious freedom: 'We urge,' he told his Soviet hosts and his fellow guests, 'all governments to respect the rights of religious believers as outlined in the United Nations Universal Declaration of Human Righs. We must hope that some day all nations (as all those who signed the Final Act of Helsinki declared) "will recognize and respect the freedom of the individual to profess and practice, alone or in community with others, religion or belief acting in accordance with the dictates of his own conscience".'

He stressed that he was neither a pacifist nor a unilateral nuclear disarmer. He urged the conference to call the peoples of the world to prayer, and to 'rededicate ourselves personally to the task of being peacemakers in God's world.' He sat down to a spontaneous standing ovation; only one other speech in the conference, the Patriarch's, was applauded in this way.

Graham took no further part in the conference but was glad when pressure by Western delegates ensured that the conference resolutions were balanced and not, as had been expected, propaganda for the Soviet view. He had let it be known that he would leave the conference if any delegate abused the United States, and when a Middle Eastern delegate began to do so, Graham removed his earphones. The chairman noticed, and exchanged notes with other members of the platform. No more anti-American invectives were heard at the conference. Many observers felt that Graham's presence and contribution upgraded the discussions and helped other Western churchmen.

That evening Billy Graham visited the Siberians in the American Embassy. The visit had been planned for the previous day but Graham's staff had a correct hunch that his desire to exclude the media would not be respected if he went at the original time. Even when Graham reached the Embassy he nearly had to cancel because for a whole hour the Vashchenkos would not agree to his condition that no photographer or television camera record their meeting. He and his aides sympathized with the Siberians: Billy had read their story right through – twice. But privacy had been pledged; the Soviet officials would never trust him again if he broke his word. He could not sacrifice the good of the many for the few; and moreover he could achieve more for the Siberians in his own way. At last, led by Timothy Chmykhalov and his mother all six agreed, and closed the curtains between their rooms and the street above which was filled by newsmen. Yet when Billy entered the basement room, having waited all this time with the Ambassador, Alex Haraszti's sharp eye noticed a new crack in the curtains, wide enough for a camera lens in the street above to catch a picture. He closed it.

They had a pastoral visit, reading the Bible and praying together. The Siberians had rather expected something dramatic from their most famous visitor; perhaps unconsciously they were like Naaman who had supposed that Elisha would 'strike his hand upon the place.' They were much disappointed and puzzled. But their story ended as happily as Naaman's, though not so quickly. Billy persisted in his efforts, and in August sent Haraszti to Moscow; Alex was there when the six finally left the Embassy for Siberia in April 1983 on the first stage of their longed-for emigration. They reached the West not realizing how much Billy Graham had helped them.

By the Thursday morning when Billy returned to Moscow airport he was spiritually invigorated: the exuberant witness of Russian Christians, despite the pressures and restrictions, had deeply impressed him. He had preached to an estimated 8,000 persons in Moscow and rejoiced that he had been able to affirm his own faith, among believers and unbelievers, more often than he had expected. They had been 'extremely receptive. I found the Soviet people, in their hunger for the word of God, the same as I have found people in every part of the world.'

He was, however, physically exhausted and had been sleeping badly, as usual when under strain.[1] The western press had followed him everywhere, almost aggressively, throughout the visit. They had been looking for the quick scoop or sensation, but he had been thinking throughout in terms of the centuries: the almost thousand years of Christianity in Russia, the mere sixty-five years of atheist rule, the long term future. At the airport he was asked by a journalist why he 'did not speak against religious repression in the Soviet Union where the government espouses atheism'.

Graham replied that he was a guest: 'This is not the time

1. 'One of the busiest schedules of my entire ministry.' Other engagements included luncheons, dinners or receptions hosted by Metropolitan Philaret, and by Archbishop Pitirim, head of the publishing department of the Patriarchate, and by the Baptist leadership. Also meetings with Academician Georgi Arbatov, head of the Institute for U.S. and Canadian studies; with Minister Vladimir Kuroyedov, president of the state committee for religious affairs, and his colleagues, especially Vladimir Fitsev; and with Yuri Zhukov, president of the Soviet Peace Committee. Graham also met Chief Rabbi Fishman, with other leaders of the Jewish community.

nor the place to discuss it.' He added that he had found more religious freedom in the Soviet Union than was commonly supposed by Americans and that thousands of churches were open.

He then touched upon the structure of the relations between church and state. Had he been less exhausted he might not have attempted this in a few words, nor used the expression 'free church', by which he meant one that is not a state church 'like the Church of England with the Queen at its head.'[1] He was referring to historical changes since 1917 but the pressmen missed the allusion and seized upon the word 'free'.

Unknown to Graham the press had already seized and twisted an answer he gave at the earlier formal press conference on the Wednesday, before going out of Moscow to visit the monastery at Zagorsk. This was a significant occasion since it gave Graham an opportunity to speak plainly on Soviet television about Christ and spiritual revival, in answer to the question, What will help bring peace to the world?

Another of the questions put to him, by a western pressman, was: Had he personally seen religious persecution since he had been in Moscow? Graham, who had only been there four and a half days, asked: 'Do you mean, have I personally witnessed any?' The newsman said, 'Yes.' Graham answered truthfully, 'No. I have not personally seen persecution.' He could not possibly discuss in this context the Siberian Six without jeopardizing his confidential diplomacy on their behalf. And he had no idea what a storm his truthful answer would raise.

At the end of the Moscow visit he flew back to Paris and London. Three days later he took part in a transatlantic television link up for the David Brinkley show and found himself assailed and denounced. He discovered that he had become the centre of violent reproach and abuse and sorrow. He was alleged to have cared nothing for the sufferings of Soviet Christians; to have been so blind or naïve that he

---

1. The Church of England is not a state church but an established church; but few outside the United Kingdom comprehend the essential difference.

could go to Moscow and see no evidence of religious persecution in the Soviet Union; and had favourably compared the freedom of religion with that in Britain. The American press came out in a rash of bitter cartoons against him. Even many of his friends with no information except press reports were puzzled and dismayed.

He came to London to receive, at the hand of Prince Philip, the 1982 Templeton Prize for Progress in Religion: $200,000 (£110,000). He had already announced that he would give it away: partly to relieve world hunger, and part for education in the third world and part for evangelism in Britain.

Faced by a rather hostile press conference, and again in New York, he could have won instant approval by revealing his confidential discussions in Moscow or by following the practice of guests who denounce the host country as soon as they have left. He kept quiet and merely set the record straight in its context. In answer to questions he contrasted the 'tremendous' religious freedom of the West with the 'measure of freedom' in the Soviet Union, and spoke of religious persecution, but so he had in Moscow. His late hosts saw that he spoke with the same voice within their borders and without, and trusted him. Significantly, the doors soon opened to East Germany and Czechoslovakia.

The Soviet press, however, misapplied his words at the airport to build him up as the man who gave America the truth about the churches being free; and claimed (as on Radio Moscow's English service) that 'Graham said he had found more religious freedom in the Soviet Union than in Britain.' Inevitably some individual Russian believers, misled by their press, or hearing by word of mouth or letter that he had sped past the crowds outside the Baptist Church, were grieved. Graham regretted any pain caused to some of these whom he had pledged himself to help.

He had done what he could. Graham said privately and publicly that he knew he was in the will of God before he went. He was even more sure while he was there. In the small hours of the Sunday morning, May 9, after his first full day in Moscow, he confided to Haraszti: 'I feel I am in the will of God and that this visit will have an effect on the fate of our two nations and possibly on the fate of mankind.'

When he returned to America, Graham was yet more certain, despite the criticism. And the day after he returned he was scheduled to give the Commencement Address at Gordon-Conwell in Massachusetts, a conservative theological seminary. To accommodate the crowds the ceremony was moved to nearby Gordon College, and 4,000 came. When Billy walked in they gave him a standing ovation. The next night, nearly half the student body and faculty at Dartmouth College in New Hampshire turned out to hear him and when he walked in he received another standing ovation. Billy began to realize it was only a minority of Americans, both conservative and liberal, who were criticizing.

In the months that followed he received evidence enough that his work bore fruit, not least in East Germany and Czechoslovakia that autumn. In March 1983 Alex Haraszti and Walter Smyth's associate, Blair Carlson, began an extended exploratory trip through the Soviet Union, visiting many cities in Russia, Siberia, Central Asia, Georgia and the Baltic states. They were received with open arms by Orthodox and Baptists, Armenians and Lutherans, and state officials in every city. Two nights before they arrived in Novosibirsk, Western Siberia, Billy Graham had been seen on television in a programme about the Conference. This gave joy to Christians. The two Team members were left in no doubt: Billy Graham, in going to Moscow in May 1982, had been in the will of God.

A second extended preaching visit to cities of the Soviet Union was already a distinct possibility for the years ahead, and another to Rumania and Bulgaria. 'Some ask, would you do it again? I most certainly would. Jesus did not say, go into countries of the western world and preach the Gospel. He said, Go into the whole world; and that includes peoples who live under the governments of other ideologies and political and economic systems.'

21

New England

'I would certainly be willing to give my time, effort and strength to such an undertaking,' wrote Billy Graham to his director of North American crusades, Sterling Huston. Huston had outlined a boldly imaginative plan to reach all New England in the spring of 1982.

New England is the only part of the United States which thinks in regional rather than state terms: it is also the greatest centre of learning and higher education. The plan had emerged after Allan Emery, president of the Billy Graham Association, and a prominent New Englander himself, had taken soundings throughout the region. It called for a four prong approach: Billy would give evangelistic lectures in the universities; his associates would conduct seven crusades in cities of the six states from Maine to Rhode Island, with Billy preaching at the concluding rallies. Then would follow an eight day Billy Graham crusade in Boston. Finally, a few weeks later, a television crusade could reach into almost every home in New England.

Billy was receiving such a stream of requests from every continent that he could have spent all his strength, and his Team's resources, in holding crusades overseas, ignoring the equally heavy stream of requests from home. Love for his own country, his desire to help the churches, and to call yet more Americans and Canadians to Christ's service throughout the world, made him reserve a part of every year for North America. Moreover, without these crusades, which usually were shown nation-wide on television later, he would have lacked the prayer support and finance which enabled him to hold crusades in lands where the church might be small and money short.

Therefore he and the Team had criss-crossed the North American continent, holding three or four or five carefully prepared crusades every year, at cities chosen for their strategic importance to a whole region.

Sometimes a crusade became front page news in the nation, as at Las Vegas in 1980, when the MGM hotel burned down, with heavy loss of life, close to where the great meeting had been held a few hours earlier, and Billy and the Team ministered to survivors and injured. Sometimes the Team returned for a second time to a city within an appreciable distance so that the one could build upon the other. Every crusade was memorable to its region, since the churches drew thousands of Christians to work together, and tens of thousands of people gathered to hear the preaching. Afterwards, in homes and offices and shops there were new disciples learning to walk with God.

The New England crusade of March and April 1982 stands out historically for the width of its range and the boldness of the strategy, and for its impact which exceeded even the expectation.

Sterling Huston allotted more directors than usual, and as they began work they sensed at once the extraordinary interest and the high degree of expectancy. 'There was an overwhelming sense that we were about to experience God at work. The people were hungry for renewal. We just couldn't do enough for the local committees. If we planned counsellor training classes in four locations in a city, the committee would want eight. They were hungry, ready to devour any training and preparation that we could offer. At Providence, Rhode Island, for example, our Team counsellor training instructors were teaching every night of the week. We were unable to have more than four class locations, but at every location there was standing room only, and we had to move to larger facilities. Over and over again, our committees requested more instruction, more assistance, more guidance. They wanted to make sure that they did absolutely nothing which would hinder the work of the Holy Spirit through the Crusade ministry in their city.'

No less than twenty-five institutions of higher education requested an evangelistic lecture by Billy Graham. The plan allowed only for five. The selection committee had a most difficult task; such was the sorrow and complaint of universities which were declined, that Billy agreed to speak at seven on 'Peace in a nuclear age.'

At Harvard he spoke twice. By common consent these lectures were the high point of his university tour. On 20 April he spoke at Harvard's John F. Kennedy School of Government, and the day following at Memorial Church.

Some had been worried that an official invitation to a famous evangelist would create dissension in the secularized, sophisticated world of Harvard. His lecture at Kennedy was given at their regular *Forum* which distinguished statesmen had addressed. Professor Peter Gomes, the Harvard university chaplain, described the lecture as 'an elegant and deeply moving *apologia pro vita sua* which won many heads and hearts.' Graham held his cautious and critical audience spellbound as he spoke frankly and humbly of the lessons learned in his pilgrimage, and of his conviction that true peace lies only in knowing Jesus Christ.

The address at Memorial Church on the following evening was the first by an evangelist since George Whitefield, more than two hundred years before. Billy was somewhat conscious that he stood before a university; some of those present wished he had preached with his old, free fervour, for which the modern student was more ready than his predecessors. As it was, Billy could sense that his listeners were open to the Gospel and 'I tried to adjust my sermon accordingly.' The programme, in the form of a Sunday service, did not allow for him to give the invitation to come forward. Chaplain Gomes, however, told Billy to give the invitation if he wished. Billy decided to keep to the original plan. More than a hundred response cards were handed in.

'Your mission was a great time for Christians here at Harvard,' wrote the assistant minister, 'and has had a real effect upon the whole university.' Yet it was only one episode in the gruelling schedule in New England, made more strenuous because the ministry in Moscow, and the visit to London to receive the Templeton prize, had to be fitted into the middle.

'While you have been in Russia,' wrote Jim Roberts, one of the chairmen, and himself a convert of an earlier crusade, 'more than 3,000 New Hampshirites have been rejoicing over the results of the Dr. John Wesley White/Billy Graham Rally and Crusade held in Manchester. We had that many people working together to make the effort a success and all of us are praising God for the results.

'There were more than 10,000 present at your May 1 afternoon Rally and 1,000 came forward. More than 1,000 also came forward during the six nights with Dr. White. How thankful we are for all of this and how grateful we are to you for including New Hampshire in your ministry. With the State population of only 800,000, you can quickly see how profound an effect all of this will have.'

To another chairman Billy wrote:

'Never before in my ministry here in the United States have I seen such a sight as in Springfield last night when people hurried forward almost before the invitation was given! Not only is there a hunger on the part of the people, but I believe the Holy Spirit has been working here in New England in an unusual way.'

The climax came in Boston, and with it the rain. The worst storm since 1906 hit Boston on the closing Sunday afternoon of the crusade, 6 June 1982, yet 19,000 went to Nickerson Field on the Boston University campus to hear Billy Graham. 'With their faces almost hidden by rainhats, raincoats and umbrellas,' recalls Sterling Huston, 'the crowds of people sat on chairs, bleachers, and even on the wet artificial turf which in some places was covered by several inches of water that had accumulated over the weekend.'

All Boston was amazed that so many should go to an open stadium when the weather forecast offered no hope of a let-up in the rain. When Billy gave the invitation nearly a thousand splashed through the mud to make a decision for Christ, and were joined by another thousand to counsel them. Rain cascaded on counsellors and enquirers during the vital first moments of follow up.

'The presence of the Holy Spirit could not have been more real in any of the previous evangelistic thrusts or awakenings in the history of New England,' wrote the crusade chairman, Lawson L. Swearingen, to Billy. 'Although I had faith to believe that New England would respond when I agreed to devote two years to this project, I could never have sensed the magnitude of the response; and now that we have experienced it I am more convinced that the awakening is real, and that some of us should devote the next few years to make the most of the possibilities.'

Prayers could not cease, nor the great reservoir of counsellors melt away, for a few weeks after the Boston crusade came the fourth stage of the New England campaign. The Houston crusade was being shown across the nation. In New England it was delayed one week and shown with shots of the Boston crusade hurriedly edited in. In September the Boston telecast itself was shown. By this means a high proportion of New England's 13 million inhabitants had heard Billy Graham in 1982, either in person or on the screen.

The television ministry was made all the more effective by the development of telephone counselling.

The Team had tried this experimentally for years, adapting the idea from the call-ins used by politicians. To find an effective way became a particular ambition of Sterling Huston, who wanted to see a narrowing of the gap between the high numbers of viewers who were moved towards commitment to Christ by a telecast, and the comparatively few who afterwards became strong Christians. He recognized that many viewers could never be adequately counselled by mail.

In May 1980, three weeks after the Indianapolis crusade, the Team set up a number in the city, with forty lines, and showed telecasts of three of the meetings. They received an encouraging 800 calls. That November, when the Reno crusade was to be carried live on three Christian networks, the Team opened 150 lines at Minneapolis. Despite the limited viewing, 15,000 people called, many of whom made the same commitment as at a crusade. After a telecast in March 1981, counsellors dealt with 7,000 telephone enquirers but were astounded to learn that 73,000 attempts were registered by the telephone company's computer.

By the time of the telecasts of the Boston crusade the Team were using 557 lines in six centres in the United States, with 4,000 trained counsellors manning the telephones. (An early experiment of having less lines and a 'call back' offer, as at

Melbourne in 1959, was dropped because few callers would give their number until trust was established.) Every time Billy Graham goes on television for three nights some 20,000 people are counselled by telephone, yet careful survey has shown that a further 40,000 may have tried and given up.

'People struggling with alcoholism, suicide, illness, adultery, abuse, marital problems, and the occult all seek spiritual help,' say the Team. 'Some receive Christ, others only talk about their problems and then hang up. Atheists, agnostics, Satan worshippers, and others call to challenge the Counsellors.' The bulk of those who call are in earnest. A telephone enquirer has chosen to watch the telecast; has had to note down the number given, then make a call at his own expense (one American Indian youth walked a mile to a pay phone to seek counsel.) 'We find,' says Huston, 'that they are much more ready to receive Christ and receive spiritual help than many who come forward at crusades. They have a real responsiveness: they want help and they trust the people the other end.' By September 1983 nearly 200,000 people had been counselled on telephone, extending Billy Graham's ministry, through modern technology, without adding a mite to his physical burden.

At the end of 1983 the telephone ministry was taken a further step again, after the crusade in Oklahoma city that October. Charlie Riggs, head of counselling and follow up, and his assistants held training sessions in 25 cities of the State of Oklahoma. When, in December, Billy Graham telecasts were shown on three nights, and the telephones began to ring, the answering counsellor would ask the caller at the end of their conversation if he or she would like someone in their city to visit the next morning. In this way the contact was quicker, local, and more personal.

Sterling Huston sums it all up. 'We have been astounded by the demand and the spiritual hunger.'

22

Germans and Czechs

On the morning of Sunday 17 October 1982 Billy Graham preached from Luther's pulpit in the City Church of Wittenberg in the German Democratic Republic (East Germany).

All the Protestant churches of Wittenberg had been invited to take part in the Lutheran worship. As Billy mounted the ornate pulpit, which makes a splash of colour in an austere church, he murmured to his interpreter: 'Is this a *youth* service? Just look at all the young people.' A high proportion of the congregation were indeed young, with eager expectant faces; nearly forty years of atheist teaching in the schools had not taken away the hunger for God.

Billy spoke on The Faith of Martin Luther. 'It was striking to hear how Billy Graham had a deep understanding of Luther,' recalls Probst Hans Treu, a Lutheran leader of Wittenberg. 'It made a great impression on the congregation and had a very direct effect upon young people.' Afterwards many were able to crowd round him and talk with him and get his autograph. In the church courtyard and in the walk round the Luther sites, escorted by the clergy and by the Burgomaster (a government official and therefore a Marxist) he talked with ordinary people. This specially pleased him because usually in East Germany his tight schedule and the hours spent in car travel limited his personal contacts to leaders.

That afternoon Billy and his Team went to Dresden. The great baroque Church of the Cross, restored after wartime bombing, was filled to the limit; the five galleries, the aisles, the wide sanctuary were packed with over 7,000 people. Once again the young predominated; an estimated 85 per cent were under twenty two. At the end of the address over a third raised their hands.

The tour in East Germany had come after four years of diplomacy by Walter Smyth, Alexander Haraszti, and John Akers in Berlin and Washington. The invitation had come from the Baptists, through their president, Manfred Sult, and general secretary, Rolf Damman. They were joined, after early hesitations, by the former state churches, the Federation of Evangelical Churches. Bishop Wollstadt of Görlitz and Chief Church Counsellor Demke, who was later elected Bishop of Magdeburg, were their principal representatives on the preparatory committee, while the Baptists seconded their secretary for home missions, Pastor Hans-Günther Sachse, to organize. They all prepared on a national basis so that the whole of East Germany became aware of Billy Graham's coming.

The government's State Secretary for Religious Affairs, Dr. Klaus Gysi, and his deputy, Chief Department Head Peter Heinrich, who were party members and Marxists, were most co-operative: without their approval and support no such tour could take place, nor could it have been filmed for television, nor the overflow sites equipped with closed circuit television.[1]

When all difficulties had been smoothed away the visit nearly had to be cancelled because in late August 1982, while in the State of Washington for the Spokane crusade, Billy had gone walking in the nearby mountains with his youngest son, Ned, and had fallen several feet from a wet rock and injured his back. The physicians, supported by the Board of the Graham Association, wanted him to take three months' sick leave. So much was at stake in East Europe that Billy declined the advice; but throughout the tour he was not in good health. Haraszti, as his personal physician when they were travelling together, insisted that he use a large car so that he could lie full length on the journeys. Large cars in the lands of the eastern bloc are generally limited to state or party officials. The use of one by Billy Graham caused a little heart burning among Christians but was necessary, as also the fact that the Team usually had to stay at hotels reserved for

1. The equipment brought in by BGEA was then donated to the Baptist unions of East Germany and Czechoslovakia.

foreigners, though at Görlitz they had the pleasure of staying at the church house at the invitation of Bishop Wollstadt.

The twelve day tour was gruelling, despite the support of Cliff Barrows, whose preaching was another highlight for the Germans. Myrtle Hall, the black singer whose glorious voice has delighted audiences at Graham crusades throughout the world, added greatly to the joy. The itinerary involved driving south from Berlin to Wittenberg, then east to Dresden, where in addition to the main service Billy Graham addressed the synod of Saxony at the invitation of Bishop Johannes Hempel. After Görlitz on the Polish border the Team drove west across the country to Magdeburg and Stendal; then north to Rostock and Stralsund on the Baltic, where, in the mediaeval Marienkirche, Bishop Horst Genke of Greifswald gave an inspiring introduction, 'Come with us to God', before Billy preached. The final four days were back in Berlin.

Apart from the burden of the preaching, and the group meetings over meals, and the private interviews with leaders of church and state, Billy Graham had an additional stress. In a communist country his every statement, whether sermon or speech, or answers at a press conference or other function, would be scrutinized, especially by Westerners, for its political meaning, even when his intention was purely religious. In East Germany, with the tensions between the two Germanies; with the precarious balance between church and state, each competing for the attention of the people – a land where the presence of Soviet forces is common knowledge – he could not hope to please everybody. He did not wish to compromise or appease but whatever he said, or did not say, would be criticized by someone. He could only follow his own goal: to preach the Gospel in season and out of season, and depend on Christ's promise: 'It is not you that speak but the Spirit of your Father who speaks in you.'

Sometimes Billy would long to relax when the schedule demanded that he give his next address. Yet whenever he mounted a pulpit he would be conscious of an extraordinary access of strength; weariness was forgotten and the power flowed. His faithful interpreter, Rheinhold Kerstan, felt the same. Kerstan, born in Berlin, had emigrated to America

171

when a young Baptist pastor. He made a most notable contribution to Billy Graham's ministry. The Germans felt that they were not listening to a foreign preacher, so close was the rapport between the two.

Many pastors had been afraid that Billy Graham would not be able to understand the problems of the ordinary believer who must live in an atheist society. The churches in East Germany have privileges denied those in other communist lands, such as retaining ownership of hospitals and social institutions, and having their own schools for training, yet no one from outside can comprehend fully the spiritual background, the trials and complexities of daily living.

Billy's reading and personal contacts, and the preparatory work and experiences of his staff, had briefed him thoroughly, and he came with a strong desire to learn. In his preaching and his conversations Billy sought to encourage. In his interviews with high officials of the state such as Horst Sindermann, president of Parliament, he pressed upon them the civic loyalty and high moral standards of the believers, as well as speaking of his own personal faith.

He brought a message of purity and peace through the Cross. Because he preached truth his words went to the heart, especially of the young. And his hearers knew instinctively that Graham's words came from the heart. 'He lived his convictions,' said Chief Departmental Head Heinrich, who travelled everywhere with the Team. 'His conduct was the witness.'

Christians had a deeper explanation. Pastor Hans-Günther Sachse, as one of the organizers of the tour, saw much of Graham, whom he had not known personally before. 'I could not help having the impression that here is a man who shows a unity of life and word. The people see that the man is behind the word. I think that this really is a radiating out power, given by the Holy Spirit.'

It reached out not only to Christians but to Marxists in their atheism. In one city a senior member of the clergy noticed how the district and civic leaders, having officially greeted Graham with flowers on his arrival at the church door, went to the seats they had reserved for themselves, though normally they would never attend a church. 'They listened to Billy Graham intently. It was obvious they were under the influence of his preaching. And when the word of God is being preached it cannot go away void and empty. One of the officials could quote Billy Graham six months later.'

Graham's eleven day visit to East Germany led men and women to faith. It drew churches together, and 'gave courage and inspiration,' reported the notable East German Lutheran evangelist Dr Paul Toaspern, 'to many ministers and lay-workers to perform their services in a way much more strongly missionary and evangelistic.' It greatly increased respect for the small Baptist denomination. It reminded government and people that the Christian churches were a powerful force for the good of the masses.

At Stendal, a small city north of Magdeburg, Billy was to preach in the evening in the 12th century Lutheran cathedral of St Nikolaus, which in effect is two churches divided by a great screen, an architectural curiosity which could be used as a pulpit on great occasions. It is reached by a very narrow twisting stairway.

Early in the afternoon a large number of young people from Stendal and surrounding cities gathered in the forecourt of the cathedral. The sight attracted others who came out of curiosity. The doors opened and the church filled up with 2,500 people, mostly young. About an hour before Billy Graham was due they started singing. The quiet Christian songs and the sight of so many worshippers was unforget-table to young and old. 'Our state officials,' recalls one of the clergy, 'were deeply impressed to see that many people, causing no disturbance, behaving decently, and come together for the sole purpose of hearing the Word of God.'

A Czechoslovakian Baptist pastor, Jan Kriska, had been an atheist in his youth. Several of his companions rose to high positions in the Communist Party and the state. He had long nourished a hope of bringing in Billy Graham for a preaching tour but his government friends laughed at the very idea. Early in 1982, however, one of them told him that after Graham's visit to Moscow they would consider him for Czechoslovakia.

In due time Kriska sent a letter which was handed to Billy in Moscow, inviting him to stop in the Czechoslovak Socialist Republic on his way home in May. He was unable to accept. After negotiations by Smyth, Haraszti and Akers with Czechoslovak officials in Washington and Prague, where Director Karel Hruja of the state office for church affairs was most helpful, a five day visit was arranged to follow East Germany.

Billy flew from Berlin (East) after a delay from bad weather and rested three days in Vienna. Here he was bought the final schedule for Czechoslovakia. When he saw it he winced.

From his arrival and press conference at Prague airport on Friday, 29 October, which was shown on state television, until his departure on the following Thursday morning his days were full to the limit of his strength.

His hosts were the Baptist Union, led by its president, Pavel Titera, and its general secretary, Stanislav Svec, who would also be his interpreter. The Baptists were one of the smaller churches; the Roman Catholic is the most numerous, and formerly exerted much political power. Lutherans and Reformed are strong in Slovakia. It had been hoped that Billy Graham's hosts would be the Ecumenical Council, on which seven other churches are represented with the Baptists, but the wider invitation did not work out on this visit. The Marxist, and thus atheist, government pays the salaries of all priests and clergy and spends money on the maintenance of church buildings, but exerts an overall control on religious activities. Billy spoke privately, and several times publicly, about the tensions which arise.

In the beautiful city of Prague, with its historic buildings, he preached on the Sunday morning in the Baptist church, where 1,200 crowded in, and in the evening at St Salvator, a seventeenth century church of the Evangelical Czech Brethren which is the largest Protestant building in Prague. Wherever he preached, tickets were issued through the churches, to prevent overcrowding. The demand exceeded the supply, and St Salvator could have absorbed considerably more than the 3,000 who listened to Billy that night. Scores who could not show a ticket were courteously turned away by the police, who would not permit them to linger outside during the service.

The Czechoslovaks loved Billy's simplicity and directness, and the little touches of humour with which he often began his addresses. In Prague, in Brno, chief city of Moravia, and at Bratislava, the city on the Danube which is capital of the Slovak republic, there were touching incidents. A hundred strong youth choir in Prague, with the men in blue suits and white shirts and the women in blue skirts and rose coloured blouses, sang contemporary Czech Christian music and then joined Myrtle Hall, who had sung spirituals, in a rousing *Amen*. In Bratislava a forty strong children's choir sang in front of the pulpit and then presented Billy and each member of the Team with a red rose.

At Brno in the Hussite Church, seventy persons came forward for counselling, so many that they had to be directed into side rooms after the service; but at Bratislava, in the modern church building of the Brethren, the twenty-five were able to kneel at the pulpit. This was the first time in Billy's ministry in a communist country that enquirers had come forward publicly during the service. Among them was a farm worker whose mother was a Christian. He had rejected faith, got into bad company and become an alcoholic. He went forward in repentance and faith. Late that night on the twenty kilometre journey home by train and bus he was singing the songs he had learned at the meeting, to the surprise of neighbours who knew him as a drunk. At home he told his chain-smoking wife. She began to cry, threw herself on her knees and prayed aloud to be freed from chain smoking. She gave her life to Christ. Both their children became Christians and the whole family was baptized together.

Though only about ten thousand people in Czechoslovakia heard Billy Graham in person, many millions heard him on television. To the joy of Christians the state television and radio were opened to the Christian gospel during Billy Graham's visit, the first time for long years. Christians wept with joy when they found that his testimony to Christ was not cut from television news. He was on television five times (unprecedented for any foreigner) including his clear statement of faith in his informal conversation with deputy prime minister, Matej Lucan.

At Lidice, in the memorial gardens on the site of the village which the Nazis had wiped out with virtually all its inhabitants, Billy laid a wreath and made a strong declaration against nuclear war. Television viewers also heard him say: 'There is no excuse for terrorism, whatever goals it may claim. There is no excuse for the oppressive domination of one nation by another. Terror breeds terror, and cruelty breeds cruelty. How can this cycle be broken? As a Christian, I believe the basic need in our world is for a radical conversion of the human heart, a conversion which God can bring, and which will replace hate with love, greed with compassion, and the lust for power with sacrificial service.'

He also laid a wreath at the Slavin monument near Bratislava. Some Czech and American Christians had been upset when this engagement was announced, because Slavin is a memorial to the Russian war dead. Then churchmen, atheist state officials and the television viewers saw the text on Graham's wreath: 'Greater love has no man than this, that a man lay down his life for his friends. (John 15:13)' Billy spoke not only of Americans and Russians who had died for the liberation of Czechoslovakia from the Nazis; he turned the occasion to the glory of God. 'Those of us who are Christians are reminded of the greatest sacrifice of all, the sacrifice of Jesus Christ who gave His life on the cross so that we might be freed from slavery of sin and death. He died not just for one individual or one nation, but that people from all nations might put their faith in Him and acknowledge Him as Lord of all. Today He commands us to turn from our selfish way of living and follow Him in loving service and witness.'

Such words had never been heard on Czech state television. Marxists might complain that 'he is putting this Jesus Christ into everything,'; but many among the young, who in Czechoslovakia were taught indifference rather than open hostility to Christ, and were left ignorant of Christianity, were listening. Requests for Bibles showed a marked increase. Christians found neighbours more willing to ask about Christ.

Billy Graham made a deep impression on the whole nation. State officials, to whom he spoke frankly about his own faith and about the problems and sufferings caused by the Marxist attitude to religion were almost as warm as his Baptist hosts in pressing him to return for a longer visit. Billy would be happy to accept if he could use larger buildings, like the Catholic Cathedrals where he had preached in Poland; and if the invitation came from a broader group of churches.

His visits in 1982 to the German Democratic Republic and to Czechoslovakia had been steps on the way towards better understanding by Western Christians of the difficulties of their Eastern brethren; and towards a deeper respect by Marxist governments for the convictions of Christians. As for Billy, a comment by the Czech Baptist leader, Pavel Titera, sums him up: 'According to our opinion, Billy Graham is a sincere man of God from the top of his hat, and he has won our hearts for himself for ever.'

23

Amsterdam '83

In the early 1980s Billy Graham found another burden weighing on his heart.

Six years after the Lausanne Congress he was in no doubt that it had been epoch making, with profound consequences to the strategies and growth of the Christian church throughout the world. Yet neither Lausanne, nor Berlin eight years earlier, nor the regional congresses. nor the conference at Pattaya in Thailand four years after Lausanne, had been quite what Billy had intended when he had first thought up the idea in the far off days of the late nineteen-fifties.

The congresses had done much to define and strengthen evangelism but they had been meeting points for leaders, for staff officers and generals of the Christian churches rather than for the foot soldiers on whom all depended. Billy thought continually of men and women, mostly unknown, who, like the Apostle Paul and Timothy, did 'the work of an evangelist', often enduring hardship and poverty and sometimes persecution: those who pushed bicycles through jungle trails to proclaim Christ from place to place; or held missions in dense urban areas at the invitation of churches; or used other means.

Billy had no idea how many there were but he determined to hold an international conference to help them. It would be specifically for *itinerant* evangelists, since otherwise any local pastor who counted himself an evangelist might expect to be asked. Never in church history had there been an international conference of evangelists.

It would be sponsored and organized by the Billy Graham Association, who would also raise funds; every participant would pay at least part of his expenses, and some would pay all, but no one would be kept away by the cost of travel. Billy asked Walter Smyth to be executive chairman. They chose Amsterdam for its excellent communications and facilities, and because hardly a country in the world would withhold visas from citizens whose destination was Holland.

They set the date for ten days in July 1983. Billy appointed Werner Burklin as director, a West German who had worked for Youth for Christ and for the Team on both sides of the Atlantic. Werner built up an international staff of men and women with different skills and backgrounds, 'competent and above all spiritually motivated. To everyone I hired I said, "As the staff goes, so will the conference." And I was convinced that everyone had to live a holy life, not only in the office but off working hours.'

Werner Burklin, on his own initiative, travelled all over the world to explain to Church leaders the kind of men and women who were intended to be participants. He knew that in some countries the leadership would expect to nominate themselves or their relations or the usual conference hoppers; in other countries no younger person would dare to apply if older men wished to go, or even if they had declined. But Werner's explanations opened the eyes of local leadership to Billy's vision, and news of the coming conference spread quickly into the remoter areas of lands far distant from Amsterdam. Billy had laid down that 70 per cent of the participants should come from the Third World, and a good proportion be under forty.

Unlike Lausanne, where the participants were nominated by committees in their own countries, the Amsterdam secretariat made the final decision on every invitation after sifting advice from handpicked screening committees: this ensured that each participant came as an individual rather than to balance a delegation or represent a viewpoint. Originally Billy had planned for 2,500 but applications poured in, and continued to arrive even after the conference began, totalling 11,000. The secretariat found it heart breaking to refuse suitable applicants when the conference was already full: even the smoothest arrangements could not handle too big a number if the purposes were to be fulfilled. The final figure was almost 4,000. Yet, to the last moment, the staff did not know if every air ticket had reached its destination, or whether participants from more distant corners would negotiate the hazards of travel or local regulations to arrive on time.

On the broiling hot evening of Saturday 12 July 1983 the International Conference of Itinerant Evangelists, *Amsterdam 83*, opened in the great hall of the RAI centre. As the organ played, a citizen of every country which was represented brought his national flag to the platform in a colourful procession. Flag after flag came by, an impressive witness of the spread of the Christian church, until 132 flags were on parade. That evening, after the ceremonies of welcome, Billy Graham gave the key note address: *The Evangelist in a Torn World*, the first of five addresses, including a question and answer session, which he gave in the ten days. Well known names from east and west also spoke at the plenary sessions, which were interpreted into nine languages, and at the workshops in the middle of the day, when the participants separated into smaller groups according to language and interests.

From the start, Amsterdam 83 proved to be a most happy conference. Lausanne, struggling with mighty issues, inevitably had its tensions which were absent from Amsterdam where the atmosphere immediately became relaxed and joyous. Most of the participants had never travelled outside their own countries; they delighted to share and pray with kindred spirits from other lands, and to discover that their problems and pressures were not peculiar to themselves. Many had never seen more than a few hundred Christians together; now they could sing, pray and listen with thousands. Many had suffered from lack of spiritual counsel; Amsterdam provided trained counsellors to whom they could unburden in confidence. And all along, in the broiling heat wave, they were learning fresh methods and finding better ways, or contributing their own hard won experience. Nor were practical needs forgotten. Evangelists from the Third World were given cassette-players; also a parcel of clothing for themselves and their families provided by Dutch Christians and administered by Samaritan's Purse, the relief organization headed by Franklin Graham, Billy's elder son.

Billy himself was in effect the conference's host for the whole ten days. At Lausanne he had deliberately kept in the back-ground. At Amsterdam he was on the platform, with Cliff Barrows and Bev Shea, and introduced the speakers and shared his knowledge and memories. The affection of five continents flowed towards him from the massed participants, not least those from eastern Europe, who included two Orthodox Metropolitans from the Soviet Union. The East Germans were delighted to see him relaxed and in good health. 'Graham in Amsterdam was more mobile, active, joyful, free than he was in our country.'

The conference ended after ten days with a great service of Holy Communion conducted by the Bishop of Norwich from England, when the 4,000 participants and the stewards and staff took the wine together. Previously they had read aloud in unison the fifteen Amsterdam Affirmations: a small committee had worked long hours to draw up Affirmations which would express the heart of the conference and provide a non-binding code of belief and conduct. Thus the thousands who were present had words in which to rededicate themselves to the proclamation of the Gospel by life and lip in the power of the Holy Spirit, and to the building up of the Church. 'We share Christ's deep concern,' ran the fourteenth Affirmation, 'for the personal and social sufferings of humanity, and we accept our responsibility as Christians and as evangelists to do our utmost to alleviate human need.' The fifteenth and last called on the Whole Body of Christ to join in prayer and work for peace, for revival and evangelism and for 'the oneness of believers in Christ for the fulfilment of the Great Commission, until Christ returns.'

Amsterdam had reaffirmed, as Billy Graham put it in his final address, 'that while the social needs of man call for our urgent attention, we believe that ultimately these needs can be met only in and through the Gospel. Man's basic need is to be born from above – to be converted to Christ. Man must be changed. Man's biggest problem is man himself.'

Amsterdam 83 did not end when the participants scattered to the four corners of the earth to put into practice what they had learned. Billy appointed John Corts from his Team to head a follow up office based on Amsterdam. During the Conference, as John wrote: 'We saw so many opportunities, so many needs of evangelists that would break your heart.' The Association wanted to be a catalyst to make the needs known and to help supply them. A worldwide Fellowship of Itinerant Evangelists would form a loose link: membership would probably grow to some 40,000. Plans were already forming for a second conference, since Amsterdam 83 had been unable to take all who applied and should have been there. The follow up office would promote the high standards of personal and vocational life which the conference had emphasized, and would act as a clearing house for fresh ideas.

The possibilities were as limitless as the need. In whatever way the next few years might shape in detail, Billy Graham had sent a surge of encouragement across the world. He had strengthened the rising generation. Helped by hundreds, from famous speaker to humblest youthful steward, he had been the human agent in a spiritual renewal which only the future can measure.

24

Mission England

England has always had a special place in Billy Graham's affections. Following his crusades of the mid-nineteen-sixties at Earls Court in London, many had hoped to see him return. In 1968 a plan was discussed at a very high level to invite him as missioner of all the churches, including Roman Catholic, and though this did not happen, it sparked off The Call to the North, a break-through in bringing Christians together for local mission in the northern province.

In the early 'seventies Billy came for *Spre-e*[1], a youth training week organized by his Association, and for several public addresses. Then in 1975 a meeting in London, chaired by Lord Luke, debated the possibility of another Earls Court crusade. The subsequent consultations, including a session chaired by the then Archbishop of Canterbury, Donald Coggan, produced the Nationwide Initiative in Evangelism, but no crusade. Billy was determined not to obtrude himself; he had a full programme in other parts of the world to the limit of his physical resources.

In November 1978 an Anglican clergyman in his early forties, Gavin Reid, wrote a widely quoted article in a church weekly. Reid's work was in evangelism and church growth. He had never forgotten how he had gone for his first curacy to a dockers' parish in the east end of London, five years after Harringay. He had found his next door neighbour to be a Harringay convert, and the door beyond, and three doors up: 'I am totally convinced about Billy's ministry because I was in a parish full of Billy Graham converts.' In his article Reid deplored that three years of consultation had led nowhere. He urged bringing Billy back to Britain before the initiative was lost.

The following February, 1979, the *Guardian* newspaper published an article by a clergyman headed, 'Stay Away Billy

1. *Spre-e*: '*Spiritual Re-emphasis*'.

Graham,' which also attacked David Watson, the well known Anglican evangelist. Reaction by readers obliged the *Guardian* to run a second article, by a clergyman who defended Watson and wanted Billy back. The BBC broadcast a debate by the two men and invited listeners to vote by postcard. The result astonished the BBC who announced on 4 March: out of 14,991 cards received, 13,825 wrote 'Billy Graham *Yes*,' and only 1,166 wrote 'Billy Graham *No*'.

The Council of the Evangelical Alliance then cabled Billy Graham an invitation to hold another crusade. Five days later an unrelated private group, from many cities, met in Birmingham and sent a similar invitation, having 'lost patience with the consultative procedures.' Walter Smyth brought the two initiatives together but Billy decided to reserve judgement because he had already agreed to preach at Oxford and Cambridge early in 1980. The Christian Union at Cambridge University had secured him as their triennial missioner, twenty-five years after his famous mission of 1955; and Michael Green, rector of St Aldate's, Oxford, which is surrounded by colleges, had asked him to come first to Oxford for a four day mission to town and gown.

'I carry a special burden in my heart for students', Billy wrote, knowing the need to reach them with the Gospel in the years when they decide the direction of their lives. The importance of Oxford and Cambridge made him hope for a preparation period of reading and thought, free of too many engagements, but the great student conference at Urbana, plus a string of television opportunities and a Methodist church conference on evangelism left little time. On arrival in England he slipped in the hotel bathroom and fractured several ribs.

Throughout Oxford, therefore, Billy was in pain, and suffering a touch of pleurisy, as he preached at the meetings in the Town Hall and as he addressed the Oxford Union Debating Society, a forum which has heard many famous figures down the years. He feels in retrospect his addresses lacked the freshness of those he gave at Harvard two years later; moreover the audience at the mission was mixed between townsfolk of all ages and university students, yet each required a different approach in a setting so intimate as Oxford Town Hall: the problem would not have arisen in a stadium.

The Oxford churches were greatly encouraged, with many new converts to join their carefully prepared nurture groups. The British press gave Billy Graham attention which no other foreign religious leader received until the coming of the Pope. Some reporters still approached Billy cynically or with tongue-in-cheek. Their pieces read almost as if they had looked up what their paper had written in 1954 before Harringay, but never read on to discover the profound change of attitude in the British press, nor researched his development and achievement since. They seemed puzzled that Graham was different from preconceptions. But he made Christianity news.

At Cambridge the student audience in Great St Mary's, the university church, filled every seat nearly an hour before each service. A body calling itself Students Against Mass Indoctrination (SAMI) had helped to stir up interest in advance; however, their assertions about Billy's character, methods and message were so wide of the mark that SAMI melted away once he had arrived. The entire university talked about the mission; Graham was the topic in halls and lecture rooms and wherever undergraduates met. Every college had received an assistant missioner, and the Christian Union had prepared thoroughly. Billy sought to do whatever the executive of young men and women advised, which somewhat astonished them. He believed that many more students would have responded at the end of each sermon had he given an invitation, but the executive were sure that coming forward was not the way to lasting decisions, in the Cambridge of 1980.

Billy was delighted at his audiences, who warmed to him and listened closely. The mission of 1955 had begun in controversy with a long correspondence in *The Times* but that of 1980 was a happy mission; 'I felt the interest was far deeper than it had been when I was here 25 years ago.' Billy delayed his departure by one day to meet Christians, whether new or established, in Holy Trinity church. The

185

vicar, Michael Rees, found the church so full that he sat on his vestry steps. 'Following a simple challenge to "full-time" Christian work at home or abroad,' he wrote, 'Dr Graham asked those who were prepared to serve God in this way to stand. The building virtually stood. The results? Eternity alone will tell, but it could well be that we shall see an upsurge of men and women coming forward for dedicated Christian work over the next five years as a direct result of this mission.'

A university mission cannot be assessed or written about in detail for many years. Out of 1955 had come the 'Cambridge Seventy,' and leaders such as Michael Cassidy. Billy was encouraged when the newly appointed Archbishop of Canterbury, Robert Runcie, spoke of the 1955 mission and that he had been impressed by Graham's perception of the students.

It was when Billy returned to England to be a guest at the new archbishop's enthronement that he attended a meeting in London arranged by the Evangelical Alliance on 24 March 1980, which handed him a formal request with a hundred signatures to hold another crusade. The sixty four signatories present included the Bishop of Norwich and many clergy in strongly active parishes or districts; also a Member of Parliament and a retired MP, and the recently retired Chief of the Defence Staff. Billy and Ruth came straight from lunching with the Queen.

An incident at this meeting in the hall below All Souls' Church, Langham Place, next door to Broadcasting House, proved to be the vital link in the chain. The chairman, Gilbert Kirby, asked whether any one too young to remember Harringay might wish to add a question. His own son-in-law, Clive Calver, who had been converted off the streets of the east end of London and had put new force and fire into Youth for Christ, respectfully asked why so few of the signatories were under forty, since two-thirds of the attendance at any crusade would be under forty. Afterwards Billy and Walter buttonholed Clive to ask about these younger leaders of whom he spoke, and of the surge of Christian conviction among the young. They challenged him to bring some of them together to meet Walter.

Clive brought twenty-three to a small London hotel on 29 March. They were similar in age to the group which had mounted the Harringay crusade when Billy Graham was thirty-five years old. As a result it was agreed that at least half of any crusade executive would be under forty years of age.

That same evening Walter Smyth met older evangelicals, and conveyed a personal request from Billy for a small steering committee: five older, five younger, together with Walter Smyth and Maurice Rowlandson, Billy's London director and personal representative in Britain. The twelve met and sketched out a plan a month later.

Billy did not hurry to decide. One of his gifts is a sense of timing. Singapore, for instance, had begged again and again for a crusade; Billy felt that the time was not ripe. Then a revival swept through churches and their leaders, including the Anglican bishop, with the result that the Billy Graham crusade of December 1978 made a tremendous and lasting impact on Singapore and the churches were thoroughly prepared to follow up.

Consultations in 1980 convinced Graham that England was not ready. He would have strong yet only sectional support. Many church leaders still believed that 'campaign evangelism' would dampen rather than strengthen parish evangelism, despite evidence to the contrary from Sydney, America, Singapore and elsewhere. While he began his crusades in Japan in October, therefore, his friends in England had to digest a letter conveying a qualified *No*: he might come but not yet.

In January 1981, after his second visit to Poland and Hungary and his private meeting with the Pope, Billy Graham was again in England for a debate with Lord Ramsey of Canterbury, the former archbishop, at Great St Mary's, Cambridge. In London Billy was begged to reconsider his decision. He replied: 'Why don't you call together the little group who put up a plan, and have another look at it?'

So they met at the Mission to Lepers to plan a mission to England. They found their earlier suggestions to be sound in substance. The hour was late and England more than ever a mission field needing a clear, resounding proclamation of Christ and his cross. They were sure that Billy Graham was the only man on earth who could bring the English churches together for mission and command the nation's attention. At the time of the meeting the rescue of the missionary hostages in Iran was much in the news: long fruitless negotiations had been resolved when the Archbishop of Canterbury's representative flew out to Iran. Gavin Reid exclaimed: 'We will never get anywhere by correspondence. Let's put up the money and fly to America.'

They found that Billy was coming to Europe in the summer. Early in July 1981, therefore, Gavin Reid, Clive Calver, and Eddie Gibbs of the Bible Society, together with David Rennie, chairman of the Billy Graham Association's London Board, and Maurice Rowlandson, flew for the day to the south of France. In a basement room in a hotel at Nice, sadly without a view of the sea, they opened their plan to Billy.

They wanted a three year 'Mission to England with Billy Graham'. The first year would be for prayer, local evangelism and thorough preparation by the churches. During the second, Billy would preach at missions, eight days long, in different regions of England except London, using the football stadiums of strategically placed cities. The effect would be cumulative, right across the nation. (A mission to London with Luis Palau was already being planned independently). The third year would not merely follow up converts: the Billy Graham missions would be the launching pads of an even wider evangelism, in market towns, in cities and the countryside, as each diocese and district made the most, under God, of the interest and spiritual hunger and the flood of new converts eager to pass on their faith.

'We cannot guarantee to deliver anything to you,' the three told Billy, 'but we think we can. People are doubting whether you will ever come, and the only way to break the logjam is to say we have spoken to you and we know you are willing to come if – We would like you to blank out some dates in your diary for 1984 so that we can actually say that

Billy is willing to come, and that it will be the summer of 1984, *if*—'

The '*if*' was that the churches understood that he was not coming to do a crusade in itself like Harringay or Earls Court but to share a three year, open-ended endeavour by them all, and that they really wanted him.

Billy replied: 'You are asking me to come and do something *for* you, and I am not sure whether that would be right. If you are asking me to come in and do something *with* you, I find that very exciting.' He agreed, exceptionally, to hold open an entire three months until they could test the response.

During the autumn of 1981 the plan was put to each region. Originally they had proposed three; this grew to five. The meetings were public and widely advertised, a genuine sounding of opinion. All five responded favourably. A change of mood was plainly taking place. Calls and initiatives had come and gone, leaving scarcely a ripple. Christians now wanted a campaign, provided it were like Mission England, and few doubted that Billy Graham was the only evangelist who could catch the ear of the nation. A little incident at Norwich was a token of what might happen. When the speakers were lunching after the meeting they were interrupted by their waitress. 'Do you mind if I say something?' They looked up surprised. 'I do hope Dr Graham comes back. Because twenty years ago it was he who er . . . well . . . brought me to God!'

Despite the favourable response; Billy did not give immediate acceptance. Then he went to Blackpool in the last days of February 1982 – the time when he was deciding finally about Moscow – to address the Christian Booksellers conference.

He had accepted the invitation because of the affection of the whole Team for the conference secretary, Jean Wilson, formerly of his London office. Once it was announced that he would be coming, West Lancashire Christians had begged that he stay on for a mini-crusade. The thorough preparations, size, warmth and affection of his audience at the two rallies, and the high response to his closing invitations to decide for Christ, moved Billy Graham

189

profoundly. The local press gave generous coverage, commenting that he had drawn the largest audiences in the town's history. Although, said one paper, there were other famous evangelists in America, 'none is more welcome on this side of the Atlantic than Dr Graham himself. His message to mankind does not change and is so simple that a child can understand it.'

After Blackpool Billy went to a private meeting at Manchester of clergy and laity drawn from the five proposed regions. The title 'Mission England' was proposed and adopted to cover the entire three year concept. A formal invitation was drafted, typed out, signed by all present and given to Billy Graham. He had no further hesitation. Within a few weeks he sent his acceptance for the summer of 1984.

The concept caught on at once. In one region which was not originally included in Billy Graham's schedules, the three diocesan bishops had approached the Mission England office and secured a change of plan. Another bishop whose diocese was not well placed geographically for the stadium chosen for that region, tried to get his city included, but the schedule was now as full as Billy's strength would allow.[1]

The time was ripe. A new spirit was stirring in the nation, a new hope and sense of purpose. The courage and sacrifices of the war in the South Atlantic crystalised a widespread desire to return to Christian values. All over the country men and women were recognizing the emptiness of materialism and, as a leading article in *The Times* put it in January 1983, that 'A society tuned only on a secular scale is unstable. It is shorn of its spiritual substance.' They repudiated the permissiveness and self-seeking of the past twenty years which had sapped the national charater. They looked for deeper answers to the fearsome problems and anxieties of the age. Ears and hearts were open again to the message of Christ.

During 1983 the preliminary rallies and preparations for Mission England were already bearing fruit. Local leaders,

1. *South-west*: Bristol; *North-east*: Sunderland; *Midlands*: Birmingham; *North-west*: Liverpool; *East Anglia*: Norwich and Ipswich.

a small central office, and members of the Billy Graham Team all worked closely together and many imaginative plans were afoot, such as videos carried by datapost, spreading the stadium meetings far and wide. There was a rising expectation that Mission England would indeed turn a page in history and make evangelism a feature of the end of the twentieth century. 'What we long to see' said Walter Smyth, 'is that this mission – six centres but one mission – should be the beginning of spiritual renewal throughout Great Britain.'

On 8 November 1983 Billy Graham celebrated his 65th birthday. Earlier in the year President Reagan had presented him with America's highest civil award, the Presidential Medal of Freedom. On the actual birthday the city and county of Los Angeles invited him to unveil a plaque at the corner of Washington and Hill Streets, on a civic building opposite the site of the tent where he had preached in 1949 and had sprung to fame. With him were Cliff Barrows, Bev Shea and others of the Team who had worked with him ever since: one of Billy Graham's strengths has been the Christian testimony of a Team whose principals have stayed together, growing and deepening and enduring for nearly forty years.

Early in 1984 Billy came to England for two crowded weeks. He addressed 11,800 ministers who converged on Birmingham from all the regions, despite snow: a most inspiring occasion. In London, at Lambeth Palace, the Archbishop of Canterbury hosted a reception for Billy Graham, with fifty church leaders, drawn from every denomination; Billy was encouraged by their willingness. The Archbishop gave a very warm welcome to Graham, giving three reasons why he was glad to do so and to support him for Mission England. At 10 Downing Street Billy Graham had a private discussion with the Prime Minister. He also had a meeting with the Lord Mayor, Dame Mary Donaldson, and other private engagements and numerous newspaper, television and radio interviews.

Billy and Ruth were house-guests in Norfolk of Her Majesty the Queen and the Duke of Edinburgh, and Queen Elizabeth the Queen Mother. For many in the land, Mission

191

England's year with Billy Graham seemed truly to begin when he preached at the Sunday morning service in Sandringham parish church.

The Royal Family sit in the chancel. The nave of the little village church holds only 115 people, with the robed choir, and all were either members of the royal household or parishioners or their house-guests. The rector, Gerry Murphy, had visited every family in his group of parishes the previous week, and some came who seldom went to church. The congregation was the nation in miniature: the Sovereign and her subjects. In the park, even though it was snowing fourteen miles away, over 2,000 people stood outside in the bitter cold listening to the entire service by loudspeaker.

The hymns and lessons focussed on the Good Shepherd. Then Billy mounted the ornate pulpit of oak and silver, gift of an American millionaire in memory of King Edward VII. Behind Billy stood a silver processional cross, 400 years old. Above him was the bas-relief portrait memorial to King George V.

After delighting the entire congregation with a bit of humour, he preached on the Twenty Third psalm, which had been sung earlier to *Crimond*. Speaking quite fast he gave a simple, strong message of hope, for he showed how the Good Shepherd meets the human problems of sin, suffering, death, and the future. Everyone is searching for purpose and meaning in their lives. Their souls needed to be restored to God. 'God is saying from the cross, "I love you. Turn to Me and I will solve your problems." '

Billy Graham that Sunday morning preached the eternal Gospel. He had preached it in 65 countries and, in God's good time would preach it in all the regions of England that summer. As he said after the service, standing in Sandringham churchyard before the millions who would watch on television news: 'My job is to be faithful, to proclaim the Gospel wherever I am . . . It is always a time of tremendous soul searching for me, and a great privilege, with a sense of humility and unworthiness, to preach the Gospel at anytime.'